THE
STILLNESS
OF LIFE

THE STILLNESS OF LIFE

The Osteopathic Philosophy of
ROLLIN E. BECKER, D.O.

Edited by Rachel E. Brooks, M.D.

STILLNESS PRESS

Stillness Press, LLC.
PO Box 18054
Portland, OR 97218
Phone/Fax: 1-503-265-5002

Edited by Rachel E. Brooks, M.D.
Book and jacket design by Lubosh Cech

ISBN 0-9675851-1-2

For ordering information see p. 273.

To Don and Ginny Becker

CONTENTS

Preface *xi*
Introduction *xv*

PREFACE

THE STILLNESS OF LIFE is the second volume of Dr. Rollin E. Becker's work serves as a companion to the previously published *Life in Motion*. While that first volume largely contains material Dr. Becker presented in public, this work mainly contains his more personal communication.

In this book, there is a broad range of discussion on osteopathic subjects. On one end of the spectrum are thoughtful articulations of basic concepts as Dr. Becker instructs his son during the early stages of his son's medical practice. On the other end are Dr. Becker's attempts to put into words the indescribable energetic and spiritual aspects of his understanding. He articulated some of these thoughts in public forums, but some were expressed only in personal conversations, or were expressed on paper in private correspondence and in personal musings.

During one of my visits with Dr. Becker after his retirement, we discussed the things he had chosen not to talk about publicly. I asked him specifically whether he thought the time had come when those ideas could be brought out. He answered that he did, and gave me permission to do so.

The items in this book date from 1949 to 1987. With some exceptions, the material is presented in a reverse chronological order. The material is organized in this way in the belief that where Dr. Becker's ideas ended up is the best place to start for those who would follow him. However, his earlier communications contain important features. They show the development of his ideas, helping us to understand the later versions, and they show his strong commitment to continual observation and reflection. Also revealed are concepts that he later dropped—some because he came to believe they were wrong, others because he felt he could not communicate them adequately.

Likewise, there are terms in this material that rarely appear in his public work. Some, such as "power source," seem to have been abandoned; others, such as "Silent Partner," were largely reserved for private use.

No *one* thought in this book is intended to be taken as *the* truth. Each thought should be considered in its context. Some words, such as "stillness" and "cause," are used with different meaning at different times. It is hoped that the reader will read the whole and appreciate where each thought came from and ponder where each thought took Dr. Becker and might take us now.

Most of the material in this book was extensively edited for clarity and conciseness. The goal was to maintain Dr. Becker's unique communication style while improving readability. Every effort was made to preserve his meaning, and when any uncertainty on my part existed, I left the ambiguity for the reader to consider. One exception to the editing approach is the article "A Concept for Health, Trauma, and Disease." Dr. Becker wrote this essentially for his own use, and I made only minor grammatical changes.

In this book, Dr. Becker's written correspondence, which includes letters to W.G. Sutherland and various colleagues, was handled in the following way. The letters were heavily edited to remove personal and less relevant passages. In addition, some of Dr. Becker's words were altered and grammatical changes were made. However, his basic writing style was largely left intact—preserving his use of capital letters and other such features. Ellipsis points (...), indicating material removed, were used only in those places where it seemed important for the reader to know that words or paragraphs were left out.

Copies of the original correspondence between Dr. Becker and Dr. Sutherland, as well as many other papers used as source material for this book, are in the archives of the University of North Texas Health Science Center—Texas College of Osteopathic Medicine. A number of items in this book were published over the past three years in the newsletter of The Cranial Academy; most have been edited further since appearing there. Considerable effort was made to reference and credit all quoted material, but this was often not possible.

I gratefully wish to acknowledge the enormous effort volunteered by Pat Tarzian. Her collaboration in this project has been one of sharing the joy inherent in working with Dr. Becker's words, keeping that work from ever feeling burdensome by taking on endless tasks, and helping his words to come alive.

My deepest thanks go to my teachers, Swami Chetanananda and Rollin Becker. The great kinship and respect they had for each other created an extraordinary path for me to travel, and they inspire all my work. These feelings are captured in a dedication Chetanananda inscribed: "...to Dr. Rollin E. Becker, whose life work we hold in the highest regard. He served humanity deeply by demonstrating the healing potential in Dynamic Stillness."

INTRODUCTION

ROLLIN E. BECKER strongly believed that a philosophy, no matter how great it might sound, was of little use unless it had a practical expression. Given this belief, osteopathy was a perfect venue for Dr. Becker's life work. Osteopathy's philosophy is far-reaching, and its application to patient care is direct. Osteopathic understanding, as enunciated by its founder, Andrew Taylor Still, encompasses everything from the physical structure of the body to the universal forces that govern all nature. Similarly, the practice of osteopathy has within it the simple taking hold of a bone as well as being conscious of all the forces operating in the patient, including his or her highest spiritual nature.

Dr. Becker found this all-encompassing approach to osteopathy demonstrated in a living way in William G. Sutherland, D.O. Not long before they met, Dr. Becker had made a commitment to himself to learn more about osteopathy—the laws that govern nature and the practical application of them to help mankind. He became a dedicated student of Dr. Sutherland, and a close personal relationship developed between teacher and student during the last decade of Dr. Sutherland's life.

After Dr. Sutherland's death in 1954, Dr. Becker, together with a small group of other osteopaths, persevered in keeping Dr. Sutherland's teaching alive. Perseverance was needed, as they found little professional interest or support for this expansion of osteopathic understanding into the cranial field. It is difficult today to appreciate how close osteopathy in the cranial field came to being lost in the years after Dr. Sutherland's death.

I believe that this lack of an open and receptive forum contributed to the reluctance Dr. Becker had to speaking all his thoughts in public. In his attempts to communicate his thinking to the profession, his experience was that his ideas either were discounted or were not understood. While he never doubted his own thinking, based as it was on his own observations and clinical results, he did doubt his capacity to communicate it to others. Dr. Becker minded less that people would discount what he said than that they would misinterpret or misuse the information. When he failed to get his meaning across to others, he assumed the limitation was largely his own. Even in those instances when other physicians appeared to understand what he was saying, he found few who were interested in deeply pursuing the work for themselves.

Dr. Becker's reluctance to express his ideas probably was also influenced by Dr. Sutherland's philosophy of teaching. According to Anne Wales, D.O., another one of Dr. Sutherland's students, Dr. Sutherland, when teaching, would say only what he believed the audience was ready to hear. His goal was to give each audience the next piece of information they needed to continue their progress in this work. He would suggest the possibilities that lay ahead, but these were often in the form of allusions, and the interested student needed to read between the lines. Given this strategy, it was often the case that Dr. Sutherland said one thing in public forums and another thing in his private interactions with each of his close students. Similarly, Dr. Becker was cautious about presenting concepts he believed students were not prepared to understand.

As I stated in the introduction to *Life in Motion*:

Osteopathy in Dr. Becker's hands focused on "Life in motion" and Stillness....While recognizing that life manifests as motion, he also understood that the power of life resides in Stillness....All life springs forth from this power, and the nature of this power is stillness—a dynamic stillness full of potential and a stillness that one can learn to palpate as surely as one can palpate motion. These properties of life, motion, potency, and stillness are all available resources in the restoration of health. (p. xviii)

In most teaching venues, Dr. Becker emphasized motion more than stillness, as the concept of motion and the skills required to use it are more easily grasped. In his own thinking and in his private communication, however, he emphasized stillness.

Another reason for Dr. Becker's emphasis on motion in his teaching was his belief that each new level of understanding is built upon and integrated with the knowledge one already has. In embracing the concept of stillness and all that it implies, Dr. Becker never diminished the value of all he had learned before. He never spoke of leaving behind a given skill; instead he continually worked to refine its use. His teaching started with the basics, as that is where even the most gifted student must begin and become accomplished. Like Dr. Sutherland, however, he also tried to point in the direction of the knowledge and skills that lay ahead.

Dr. Becker was also influenced by Dr. Sutherland's pragmatic view of what was appropriate for a given time. In a 1950 letter to Dr. Becker, Dr. Sutherland wrote, ..."It [is] important at this stage to keep clear of the spiritual....It is necessary for the present to keep to the material [level] concerning material for publication." Dr. Becker's own experiences confirmed that discussions of spirituality often led to confused or reactionary responses.

Since the earliest days of osteopathy the question has been asked, Is osteopathy a religion? Dr. Still, the son of a Methodist minister, was asked this question, as his writings are rooted in references to God and the all-knowing Architect. Dr. Sutherland, who fully accepted Dr. Still's teachings and used biblical quotations to illustrate some of his concepts, was also asked this question. And, after reading these works of Dr. Becker, the same could be asked of him.

The question arises because each of these men expressed his firm belief that there is a vital, universal, divine force that pervades and governs the nature of all things. None of them personally maintained any connection with an organized religion, but each perceived himself and everyone else as spiritual beings. For these men, scientific reasoning and spirituality were seen as a seamless whole. In response to the question posed, they might have said that the science of osteopathy is not a religion, but it does embody all spiritual truths, as must be the case with all scientific realities. An article in *Science News* that Dr. Becker had among his papers suggests: "Perhaps what is needed is [an approach]...in which all of the methods that humanity has historically used to approach reality—scientific, philosophical, theological, aesthetic, even mystical—are used together in all of their vigor."

Dr. Becker's view of life was also strongly influenced by his parents. His father, Arthur D. Becker, was a highly respected doctor of osteopathy who served as dean of two osteopathic colleges. He began his teaching career at the American School of Osteopathy at a time when Dr. Still continued to keep a watchful eye. The senior Dr. Becker modeled for his son a thoughtful reverence for osteopathy and Dr. Still's teachings. His mother, Mabel, had deeply held spiritual beliefs, and in her conscientious effort to live her life in accordance with them, she imparted their value to her son.

Dr. Becker's personal spiritual view was that each person has, and is responsible for, his or her own one-on-one relationship with the Divine. He believed there is nothing more profound and nothing more simple than this relationship. In his life and in his practice of osteopathy, Dr. Becker strove for a total reliance on his "Silent Partner," or the "Boss," as he termed it. In a May, 1979 seminar, he said, "I love my work and am grateful for the opportunity to do it. It doesn't ultimately have anything to do with anybody else, but it's a wonderful thing to have the opportunity to be reminded to contact your Silent Partner, and to surrender again and again. This opportunity is what all the cases I see represent, and it's a good thing."

Osteopathy and the Cranial Concept

This section is reprinted from the introduction to Life in Motion.

The science of osteopathy was discovered in 1874 by Dr. Andrew Taylor Still, a medical physician ardently searching for a more effective system of healing. His intense study brought insights that led him to articulate a number of fundamental principles. He taught that the structure of the body and how it functions are inextricably linked and that each person contains within himself the resources necessary for health. He also maintained that the body is a unit of function—that body, mind, and spirit operate as a unified whole continually working to heal itself. Dr. Still conceived of all diseases and ailments as involving some impairment in the free flow of the material and energetic elements within the body, thereby impeding the self-correcting process within.

Based on an understanding of these principles, Dr. Still developed an approach which used the physician's knowledge, understanding, and hands as the primary tools in both diagnosis and treatment. The college he established taught the full array of medical and surgical knowledge, but Dr. Still's emphasis always remained on a thorough understanding of anatomy and physiology and the application of palpatory skills. Over time, various osteopathic manipulative approaches have been developed to apply these principles to the treatment of patients.

It was in 1892 that Dr. Still established the American School of Osteopathy in Kirksville, Missouri, and in the class of 1900 was a man named William Garner Sutherland. While a student at the college, Dr. Sutherland also had a flash of insight into the inherent mechanisms within the human body. He had the thought strike him that the bones of the living cranium maintain a movement throughout life which indicates the presence of a type of respiration. Through dedicated study, observation, and self-experimentation over a period of 40 years, Dr. Sutherland worked out the details of this respiratory mechanism. He then spent the last 15 years of his life teaching others this *cranial concept* and the practical application of it to patient care, which became known as *cranial osteopathy* or *osteopathy in the cranial field*. In all his teaching, Dr. Sutherland never failed to emphasize that the cranial concept was only an extension of, not apart from, Dr. Still's science of osteopathy.

Dr. Sutherland's discovery went far beyond the description of a mechanical system; he came to understand that the movement he observed is the basic life force in operation. It is a manifestation of life in motion—an outward sign of the fundamental self-regulating, self-healing mechanisms in the body.

Because of this mechanism's fundamental nature and its rhythmic quality, Dr. Sutherland termed it the *primary respiratory mechanism* (also called the *craniosacral mechanism*). He described five components of this mechanism that function as a unified whole. The five components are: 1) the fluctuation of the cerebrospinal fluid, with the potency of the tide; 2) the inherent motility of the central nervous system; 3) the mobility of the cranial and spinal dural membranes (reciprocal tension membrane); 4) the articular mobility of the cranial bones; and 5) the involuntary mobility of the sacrum between the ilia.

Having come to an understanding of the anatomy and physiology of this subtle but powerful mechanism, Dr. Sutherland was also able to establish treatment principles for working *with* this mechanism. He developed an approach, using hands-on manipulation, that was as subtle and powerful as the mechanism it was working with. Dr. Sutherland's approach to treatment can be summarized in his injunction, "Allow physiologic functioning within to manifest its own unerring potency, rather than apply blind force from without."

The understanding and approach taught by Dr. Sutherland was never limited to the cranial mechanism. This primary respiratory mechanism is represented in all of body physiology. Therefore, while it is uniquely suited to treat problems in the cranial field, it can potentially affect any situation arising from disease or trauma in the body.

1. Ann Arbor Seminar

This is an edited transcription of an informal meeting with Dr. Becker and a small group of medical students who were members of a spiritual community. The seminar took place in May 1979 in Ann Arbor, Michigan.

Biography

I've been practicing for 45 years, having graduated in 1934 as an osteopathic physician in Kirksville, Missouri. After a short stint in Oklahoma, I spent about 13 years practicing in Pontiac, Michigan, and I've been in Dallas, Texas, for the last 30 years. For the first ten years of my practice, I was in general practice, doing a little bit of everything—surgery, delivering babies, and everything else. I also used a lot of osteopathy, if you want to call it that. But then during the last four or five years that I was in Michigan, I decided that the osteopathy I had been taught to use deserved a closer look.

At the time, I had a good practice and was getting good results with the osteopathic treatments I was giving, except that it bothered me that I never knew why I was getting the results I did. I wondered why certain people did better than others. For example, if I had ten young workers with low back strain and I'd give them all my so-called osteopathic treatment, three of them would make a fantastic recovery, others would make a good recovery, and the last guy would still be struggling with it six weeks later. Why was this, if I'd given them all a good treatment? I must not have been working with the tools that were designed by the patient; instead I was working with the tools that I had been taught.

I decided there had to be a better route, and during the last five years I was in Michigan, I kept playing around with this. I kept working out ideas, going up blind alleys, backing out again when nothing happened, and then trying a different direction. Eventually, by the end of the five years, I had pretty well discovered how to begin to work. I was able to begin to understand some of the things the patient's body was telling me and was able to cooperate with it to the point where the patient's own problem was teaching me. With this approach, I found I could now begin to understand why patients were experiencing the results they were. By the time I left Michigan, I was doing the kind of treating I still do today.

For some time, I had been thinking about relocating from Michigan to Texas, but when it came down to it, the time between when I made the final decision to move and when I actually moved was just three weeks. This was a very rapid transit, to say the least, and during that three-week period, over 200 patients came to me and said, "We like what you are doing. We like the type of treatment you do now. It works better than what you used to do. We see you for a fewer number of visits, and we stay healthier between visits. We want to continue this type of treatment. Who can you send us to?" Well, there wasn't anybody. And believe it or not, that was the first time anybody had ever told me they liked what I was doing.

When I went to Texas, I didn't bother going into general practice; I don't practice "general medicine." I don't have connections with any hospitals. I don't have anything. I just have an office with a table, and I give treatments. I do not consider myself to be the patient's primary physician. I never was the primary physician anyway; I still say the patient is the primary physician. Whatever I do is supplemental to whatever other care the patients are getting. If they're going to other doctors for cancer, ingrown toenails, or whatever, my treatment is supplemental to their care. I'm assisting their body to utilize the resources available for their particular health pattern. That's the sole purpose of the treatment. The sole purpose is to arouse the total resources of the patient's own physiologic structures.

Osteopathic Principles

The basic principle that A.T. Still enunciated was that the body is a living, breathing, dynamic organism that has all the resources and capacities necessary to do what it needs, if you can get it into a physiological balance by working with it and utilizing the organism's own resources. That's it. You don't have to introduce a lot of potent entities from the outside if you can arouse the resources of the body to handle its own problems.

The so-called osteopathic treatment Dr. Still gave was simply his way of approaching the problem of teaching the body to do what it needs. The osteopathic treatment, the manipulation, was simply a matter of: Here is the body, and it has something to say to the doctor. So why not take hold of the body and play with it until you can get some kind of change in it—manipulate it in such a way that the body hears the message, takes it back into the nervous, circulatory, and lymphatic systems, and does something with it to help improve itself.

The type of treatment that Dr. Still himself used is not really known. Nobody ever wrote down what he did, and when you read his writings, he doesn't tell you. But he does give you the principles. If you want to cure anything in the human body, the only thing you have to worry about is arousing the energies and chemicals of life to be as nature designed them. It sounds simple, but what does it mean?

We can quote one paragraph by Dr. Still, and if you understand that, you will understand all that he ever said about osteopathy. In my opinion, this is his definition of osteopathy:

> I hope all who may read after my pen will see that I am fully convinced that God, of the mind of nature, has proven His ability to plan (if plan be necessary) and to make or furnish laws of self, without patterns, for the myriads of forms of animated beings; and to thoroughly equip them for the duties of life, with their engines and batteries of motor force all in action. Each part is fully armed for duty, empowered to select and appropriate to itself from the great laboratory of nature such forces as are needed to enable it to discharge the duties peculiar to its office in the economy of life. In short, that the all-knowing Architect

has cut and numbered each part to fit its place and discharge its duties in every building in animal form, while the suns, stars, moons and comets all obey the one eternal law of life and motion.[1]

Simple? Let's take a closer look. The words "I am fully convinced that God, of the mind of nature" tell us that nature has already designed the body. You don't have to worry about it; it's here. And "has proven His ability to plan, *if plan be necessary*." Think about it. If you have a state of total health, you don't need to have any plans; it just is, and plans automatically show up. They may be necessary, but you don't have to create them. They're there; the mind of nature has already designed this organism.

Then Dr. Still says, "to make or furnish laws of self without patterns." A healthy state is a state of no pattern. If you've got a pattern, you've got a strain, a disease, or a problem. If you haven't got a problem, there's no pattern. Simple? That's true for all forms of animated being, clear out to those that are furthest afield. Everything is armed for duty with its own battery, forces, juices, and everything else. Everything is in there. It's just a question of whether you, as the physician, can learn the art, not of manipulation, but the art of living palpation that will literally get in there and work with those things that are already available. That's all he's trying to say. Simple?

Here is another quotation from A.T. Still. It's the same thing all over again:

> One has said, "Life is that calm force sent forth by Deity to vivify all nature." Let us accept and act on it as true, that life is that force sent forth by the Mind of the universe to move all nature, and apply all our energies to keep that living force at peace, by retaining the house of life in good form from foundation to dome.[2]

᙮ ᙮ ᙮

---

1. A.T. Still, *Autobiography*, pp. 148–49.
2. A.T. Still, *Philosophy and Mechanical Principles*, p. 101.

Dr. Still knew about the craniosacral mechanism—his writings show he did, but he didn't explain it. Dr. William Garner Sutherland went on to work it out. In other words, Dr. Sutherland completed the anatomy and physiology for the head and sacrum as it functions along with the rest of the body. He never distinguished his work as being any different from Dr. Still's. To him, it was just more anatomy and physiology. So those of us who are attempting to follow the basic principles that Dr. Still gave us have also to include the work that Sutherland gave, if we're going to have any decent understanding of what we're playing with. It's that simple.

⤙ ⤙ ⤙

William Garner Sutherland was a quiet man, the most beautiful man I ever met. Every one of you would love him. If you saw a picture of him, it would be like falling in love with your spiritual teacher or someone very special. He just had that kind of presence.

The Primary Respiratory Mechanism

In brief, the cerebrospinal fluid has a circulation; it has to because it's formed in a cavity, and it has to get out again. In addition, it also has the law of "life and motion." This is a really key point. What we're talking about here is life and motion—life *in* motion. The movement of the cerebrospinal fluid within the body is a true fluctuation occurring ten times a minute. The tide of the ocean rolls into the shore twice a day; within the body, within this natural cavity, it's ten times a minute. Ten times a minute the cerebrospinal fluid swells and recedes rhythmically, just like the tides of the ocean. It's a fluctuation that occurs in its own right and is not caused by the movements of the other components of the primary respiratory mechanism.

The motion of the primary respiratory mechanism is an involuntary one, and it is what maintains the life in motion of health. This little, gentle exercise that every single cell of the body is getting gives that cell the chance to be in motion, to interchange with its neighbor. The life in motion of this mechanism is absolutely essential.

Question: What is the role of the central nervous system in this life force?

The central nervous system is merely the computer for the whole mechanism. It's a very large storehouse for information coming in and going out. It's receiving information from the body, processing that information to determine what the body needs, and sending information back out again. All the basic physiological centers, including those for respiration, are located in the floor of the fourth ventricle. So it's absolutely essential for that part of the nervous system to be able to freely interchange with its environment. However, there's no one part that's more important than any other.

Dr. Sutherland believed very strongly that, in terms of *quality*, the cerebrospinal fluid was probably the highest known element in the human body. He described a relationship between the "Breath of Life" and the fluctuation of the cerebrospinal fluid.[3] We have said that the fluctuation of the cerebrospinal fluid is like the tides of the ocean—not the waves, but the tides. In order to have a tide, there has to be an incoming tide, a pause-rest point, an outgoing tide, a pause-rest point, an incoming tide, and so on. At the fulcrum point—at the point where this tide changes from one direction to the other—is the point at which the Breath of Life interchanges with the cerebrospinal fluid. It then, in turn, is transmuted into the lower energies that the body needs.

It's like when they bring electrical power into a city on 44,000-volt lines, and then they dilute that down to 110 volts so we can use it. Similarly, the original Breath of Life comes in with its full potency into the cerebrospinal fluid. This is Dr. Sutherland's concept, and I'm not going to argue with him. I agree with him. I agree with him, not because I accept the words, but because I accept the experience of it.

---

3. In *Contributions of Thought*, Dr. Sutherland stated: "The human brain is a motor; the Breath of Life is a spark of ignition to the motor, something that is not material, that we cannot see" (2nd ed., p. 147). Cf. "And the Lord God formed man of the dust of the ground, and breathed into his nostrils the breath of life; and man became a living soul" (Genesis 2:7, King James Version).

When we work with the cerebrospinal fluid, we can change its balance. We can change its pattern of fluctuation. There are ways in which we can literally still the cerebrospinal fluid. We can bring it down to a still point manually. And when it is brought through a still point, there is an interchange between every single fluid and every single cell of the body. It happens in an instant. You have transmuted the total 44,000 volts into what? An experience for every single cell to take into itself and use to revitalize itself.

I've treated at least 60 cases of true nervous breakdown—I mean nervous breakdown in the literal sense; I don't mean psychologically. The central nervous systems of these patients are just wasted. These people are just dragging one foot after the other, wondering if they are going to make it to the next minute. They are totally exhausted and feel like they haven't got anything to work with. Their chief complaint is fatigue. I don't know what causes it—the word "cause," in the ordinary sense of the word, disappeared from my lexicon many years ago—but undoubtedly it is some earlier trauma. It is due either to some physical or psychological trauma or to some disease—something that literally wiped these patients out, and they didn't make a good recovery. Then they had to carry this trauma around, their battery stayed exhausted, and it forgot how to repair itself.

When you assess or measure the vitality of these patients by your sense of touch, you find that their batteries have lost their charge. In these types of patients, you can use the CV4 approach and recharge that battery. It takes about nine months for them to finally get back up to where that charge is in the central nervous system again. You achieve this by simply stilling the cerebrospinal fluid, letting it go through its still point, and you keep doing this about once a week. Finally, after about six or nine months, all of a sudden they start hanging on to the charge. Then in about three months after that, they are back to full bloom again. That's it. The charge is in the cerebrospinal fluid.

Question: Ancient philosophical texts from India would say that between the breaths—between the in-breath and the out-breath and between the out-breath and the in-breath—is the place of God. It sounds like what you are saying.

That's right. It reminds me of a tape I had of one of Dr. Sutherland's talks in which he talked about the space between the inhalation and the exhalation. I can tell you, I sweated that thing out for months, trying to translate what he said into an experience I could be aware of and use. Of course, I guess I shouldn't complain that it took me some months—it took me five years to translate Dr. Still's definition of osteopathy into a conscious experience that could be used in a palpatory way in giving treatments. To read or hear something is fine, but it takes a long time for our sensory impulses to find out what it is that is being said. The sense of touch is very stupid.

THE NATURE OF DISEASE

Question: How does the body get out of balance and allow disease to form?

That's too broad a topic to talk about here, but I can say this. Ten days ago, I caught a cold from a baby who came in. This was a child with cerebral palsy, who incidentally also had a cold, and unfortunately I was a little fatigued and caught it. If your own resources are a bit knocked down, you have an open door for anything to move in. At the same time, you also have all the resources with which to take care of it. Disease is just a chemical process that happens in the body due to vibrations from bacteria or viruses or anything else; it is straight chemistry. Those who study homeopathy and acupuncture would say the same thing.

If you have a disease that impairs the system to the point where the body can't remember how to repair itself, it will form a pattern.

Take, for example, a chronic case of malaria, tuberculosis, or typhoid. These diseases aren't around so much anymore, but in the days before antibiotics, when I was practicing, I saw that the body would eventually secure a recovery to the best of its ability. But, as a result, the person was functioning with an imprint from that illness. Every thing they did included the chronic weakened stage of this disease they had in their system. In a way, they always had a little bit of malaria; it was always sitting there. With every subsequent process, no matter what happened, there was a program saying to every cell in the body, "You have to include me, I've gotten on your back, and I'm not getting off it." The nervous system had written the pattern in.

A beautiful example of that kind of imprint from trauma occurred in a friend of mine. He was working on a skylight, the ladder broke, and he came down and literally drove his tibia upward, shattering the femur. He came to Dallas some months later, when he finally got out of the hospital. All they had been able to do for him was to take the pieces of bone and line them up, some way or another, and cast the leg. The fracture had healed, but he hobbled around when he walked. When he came to Dallas, it was 105 degrees outside, and he was wearing wool underwear because his legs were absolutely cold. He kept putting more clothes on trying to keep his legs warm.

My view of the situation was this: How many billions of messages were being sent by that shattered leg to the lumbar enlargement of the cord, saying, "I am shattered, I am shattered, I am shattered"? How many billions of messages were being sent there day after day, week after week, month after month? As a result, everything had gone into shock. The spinal cord, which gives the orders for maintaining adequate warmth or cold, went into shock. Under this constant bombardment, the nervous system finally gave up and said, "Well, this is the way it is going to be. I hear this message, and this is the way it is going to stay." So his legs stayed cold.

Well, I treated him for about three weeks, until he left town. Then he came back again, and I started in on treatment for another few weeks. I was using the approach of tuning in to the cerebrospinal fluid and the interchange with the Breath of Life. I figured that if you can interchange with the Breath of Life, the Breath of Life should certainly know how to wipe out a bunch of lousy messages in the nervous system. Every tissue in the body automatically wants to get well, if you just give it half a chance.

One day, I was using the CV4 approach on my friend, and he said, "My god, you're burning me alive." I asked what was the matter, and he said, "That spine of mine, put your hand down there." When I put my hand down in the lumbar area, it was hotter than a red-hot poker. It was pouring heat out of that lumbar area, and immediately his legs were warm, and they've been all right ever since. I have seen this same kind of thing happen in three different cases over the years. All of a sudden, the shock comes out of that lumbar enlargement of the cord— it wakes up. All of a sudden, the tens of millions of messages from trauma that got sent to that nervous system are being wiped right out.

The point I'm trying to make is that with chronic problems, your nervous system tends to write in an adaptation, saying, "If I have to live with this, this is the way it's going to be." On the other hand, if you can figure out ways, through palpatory skills or otherwise, to train that system to wake up and look underneath that adaptation, there would also be something that would say, "This is the way I really am." If you can arouse that, it will wipe off the other.

One way I understand the issue of disease patterns—that is, how a body works in relationship to some disease pattern—is that the body comes to deal with them in a certain respect. It's not simply one pattern coming along and being overlaid on the pre-existing pattern, but the body brings itself into a new state of balance. In dealing with this disease to the best of its ability, the body also has to go on and deal with the broader process of life. Simply by having to relate to and deal with the disease, the body automatically encompasses it within the pattern of its own fluctuation.

Question: Then essentially the whole body is involved in even a localized disease process?

That's right. Everything, everywhere, is totally involved.

≈ ≈ ≈

We name diseases such as mononucleosis, chicken pox, mumps, or measles, because through the centuries we've learned to define that these sets of symptoms mean thus and so. Each one of these things has a contributing factor, a given virus that is geared to produce a certain type of music. Mumps music is different from measles music, and measles music is different from chicken pox music, but in each case, it still is a clinical entity playing a tune. When the body takes that pattern into its being—and it does so into its total being—if it could handle that particular pattern in the most efficient way possible, it would simply go ahead and play the tune. It would put the needle on the record and play the whole tune. Then when it got through playing the whole tune, the record would be a clean slate. You could start all over again, and there wouldn't be any pattern left.

In other words, ideally, the body would take in the inciting agents and handle them. It would go through the whole process of the inflammation, swollen glands, and everything else, and in the end it would correct all those problems. Then, when you got through, you would be just as good as the hour before you caught the germ. This is what would happen if you could do it efficiently, if the battle could be fought out in the open. But generally speaking, what you actually have is a lot of guerrilla warfare going on in all the tissues. The whole body is involved, but the whole body is doing other things and is going to work, despite the fact that it's got this or that. People are usually insulting themselves in one way or another. They're not getting the proper rest, their nutrition is lousy, they drink too much coffee, or they're an alcoholic. So you end up with a lot of residual hang-ups left in the various cells, which keep the patient half-sick for weeks and months afterwards. That's why it takes so long to get over some of those illnesses.

Question: But do you still get over it? Is it a clean slate?

No, you still have residues hanging around there. In the days before antibiotics, I had many experiences treating patients with lobar pneumonia using osteopathic treatment, and my patients were only sick eight days. Lobar pneumonia is an eight-day illness. If you can put them to bed and help them efficiently go through the whole routine of consolidating that lung, then at the end of the eight days, everything is cleared out and they feel great. They still have to go through all the stages of the disease, the lung has to go through all its changes, but when it is done, the patients are just as healthy as they were the day before they got it, because they had the disease efficiently.

In this kind of case, it takes a treatment twice a day to keep the body geared up and engaged in the fight. I believe that if they're going to have a fight, they should have it out in the middle of the room. In this way, they get it out of the system. It is the same with cases of mononucleosis. Mononucleosis is a 30-day illness, if you can have it efficiently.

If you knew you were going to have a disease starting tomorrow morning, and you planned to spend the next five days eating properly, resting, meditating, and just making it your life's job for those five days to cure your disease, then you'd be doing a much better job than the way you'd normally handle it, wouldn't you? But it is not very practical for us, or for our patients, to do that.

Question: How about when antibiotics are introduced?

Well, that's fine. Antibiotics definitely get the patient to go through the stages of the disease process and help in getting "over it." But my own personal opinion is that I don't think that in those cases they truly get over it. I think they get an adaptation instead.

Question: Does it weaken the body because it hasn't gone through the strengthening process?

I can't answer that. But I don't think they are the same human being afterwards that they would have been if they could have gone through the process of fighting it out with the enemy in the middle of the room and cleaning it out. Having fought it out in the open, they would be healthier than if they had to go the antibiotic route.

Question: So you don't see antibiotics working as a complement to what you do?

Well, I'm sure they do. I feel very strongly that the treatment I use helps those antibiotics to behave as they're supposed to behave. I'm sure the treatment encourages the total resources of the body and the antibiotics to do their thing. My patients all use a variety of resources for their care. I no longer practice general medicine. For whatever problem the patients present, I just do my thing and send them on for any other medical care they may need.

I want to clarify one thing. As far as I'm concerned, any form of treatment that clinically gets results in a patient is legitimate. There is no treatment that is the primary treatment. I don't care if you're talking about medicine, surgery, psychology, or what have you. A patient is a patient is a patient, and whatever it takes to make him well, those are the techniques you use. If you're using medicine, that's supplemental care to make the patient well. If you're using psychological treatment, that's supplemental care to make the patient well. If you're using surgery, that's a supplemental maneuver to make the patient well.

Question: Some people look at disease as a lesson or a positive thing.

I don't believe that at all. I'm not proud because I got a cold. There's no lesson involved. I was sitting in the right place at the right time with the right internal environment, and all of a sudden, I have a stranger in my midst. Big deal.

෴ ෴ ෴

What we call a disease is the officially accepted name for something that we learn in school. It's just an official name that is given because, according to medical science, a disease is thus and so. If it has a certain pattern, it's this disease; if it has another pattern, it's some other disease, and depending on the pattern, you treat it accordingly.

However, the no-name body physiology does not have a name for that disease.[4] It only knows it has been infected or contacted, has absorbed or taken into its pattern of living something to which it is reacting. And it's going to react chemically, immunologically, and by every other means that it has in order to respond to this insult. But it's doing it purely on a no-name basis. It doesn't recognize the germ for what it is; it simply says, "Somebody hit me with a baseball bat so I'm going to strike back." It's strictly a physiologic process of being. So when we treat utilizing the no-name body physiology and permit it to do the work it wants to do at its highest level of efficiency, it doesn't follow the patterns that we learned in the books—the "official" side of the deal.

When my daughter was about three, she was awfully fussy one night and complaining about a pain in her side. The only thing I could think of was appendicitis. It was about ten o'clock at night, and I checked her pretty carefully, went to bed, and got up in the middle of the night to check her again. Finally, when I checked her the next morning, I found one lung was consolidated, so I relaxed and said, "That's great, it's lobar pneumonia." That was the year before penicillin was invented, 1945, so for most people, pneumonia was a scary disease.

But I trusted osteopathy and just went ahead and started treating her. How I treated her was purely an experiment. At the time, I was

4. "No-name body" is a term Dr. Becker introduced in his paper, "Motion—The Key to Diagnosis and Treatment" (R.E. Becker, *Life in Motion*, p. 50). There, he wrote: "In our training to become physicians, we have dissected this body.... We have given names and descriptions of function to all parts of a complex system of cells, fluids, and mechanisms of bodily parts and their motion and movements. In reality, our anatomico-physiological body has not divided itself into the many parts we know as physicians.... It has no name..."

just beginning to think about developing the approach we're talking about. I deliberately treated her solely with this approach; I didn't even invoke a test to find out how bad the illness was. And within three days, the lung was completely clear. We took her to an air show on the fourth day. But it was the following week, eight days later, that the vitality was back to normal. This taught me that lobar pneumonia is an eight-day illness. In that time, my daughter went through the whole disease process, including the red hepatization and grey hepatization stages. But she did it at the maximum level of efficiency, and she was through with it at the end of eight days.

The neighbors, of course, couldn't believe she could get over pneumonia so quickly. They all thought I was a quack and just couldn't diagnose the problem correctly. But it shows how the flow of energy as designed by nature can do the things it's supposed to do. It's a beautiful illustration of how nature would like to work if she had half a chance to do it.

ROLE OF THE PHYSICIAN

IF YOU ARE GOING to be a physician, you are going to have to lose your ego. In doing this work, you will not be a doctor anymore. There isn't a patient that comes to my office for whom I am a doctor. I'm not a physician, and I'm not a teacher. The patient is the physician and the teacher. In fact, the patient is not even the patient. The mechanism they park in my office to be worked on is the teacher and the physician. If I insist on being the teacher or the physician, I'm guessing as to what is needed. If I listen to what the patient comes in with—their words, emotions, minds, and egos—I don't have the true picture. I must go behind that to the thing that makes them tick. Then, even they disappear.

Still, the thing they come in representing as their problem wants attention. So you go ahead and take care of it. But you do so by *listening* to it. I don't have an ego anymore; this is not my treatment. I don't give treatments. The quicker we can learn to get out of the way the better. This is true not only in medicine but also in any field. If you are an engineer and want to build a bridge, you have to have an idea of how you are going to do it, but it's the bridge itself that counts. In a treatment, if you can get yourself out of the way, what you are working on has a better chance to become what it's supposed to be than if you're sitting there directing traffic.

Now all this is assuming one thing, which is that literally what you are doing is sharing the experience of a living being with the experience of another living being. I can be a teacher to this pipe I'm smoking and take it apart, because it is relatively inanimate. But if that were a human body, it would know a whole lot more of what it needed to do within itself, because it has Life.

I accept the fact that my life is individually belonging to me, and it's alive and able to respond to the needs of this particular patient. I also accept that the patient is endowed with life and alive. When I use my sense of touch, I don't lay my hands on a patient and say, "That is hard and this is soft." Instead I accept the fact that my touch is alive. I'm alive, the patient is alive, so why not make my palpation alive? I'm accepting the premise that the patient's anatomical and physiological mechanisms are a living dynamic mechanism that is in tune with all of Life. Once I have that premise, then I can get out of the road. I can respond to the patient's mechanism and experience within it something that needs to be done.

It is necessary for me to identify with this living structure-function relationship on an individualized basis for each person. The variables of human anatomy and physiology are so different from one patient to another that I can't write common rules for each one of them. One patient is long and lanky, another is short and stocky, et cetera. Each one is different and unique. But again, they are the teacher, if I can get out of the way and be in tune with the experience. They have a problem, and I have to experience that problem. I can't experience it if I'm being a teacher; I have to experience it as a student. So I am a student of anatomy and physiology for anyone that walks into the office. To be a student, you must take your ego and dump it someplace.

Question: But it's not that you actually take that problem into yourself, is it?

It's perfectly permissible to take that problem into yourself, with all the ramifications of it. It is permissible because you are not, strictly speaking, in tune with your body. I'm not in tune with my body—I'm in tune with the thing that's going ten times a minute recharging it. I tune into that and don't pay attention to the body, which is just going along for the ride.

Here is an illustration I can give you in this regard: A man is driving down the highway at 55 miles per hour and runs head-on into a car that pulls in front of him. The next day, he comes into the office and lies down on the table on his back. I slide my hands under his back, and I'm just sitting there trying to feel what's going on. I close my eyes and immediately feel as if I'm feeling right through him, and my sensation is that I'm going right up to the ceiling. It feels so real that I open my eyes to check this out and say to myself, "What is going on?" Everything looks normal, so I close my eyes again, and immediately we're going right up to the ceiling. This time, I say, "Okay, I guess I'm here for the ride. I'll just stay with it." We stay up there about ten minutes, then something happens, and it feels as if things just drift back into my hands, until it's just him lying on the table. He now feels like himself and simply has a broken wrist.

Can you analyze what went on? It's straight physics; it's nothing complicated. If we had put a bucket of water on the car seat alongside that man when he hit the other car, where would the water go? Directly towards the point of impact. So what was the water in his body doing at the time? His total fluid mechanism was driven towards the front of the car, towards the point of contact. Twenty-four hours later, when I had my hands under him, every ounce of fluid in him, the energy in him, was going right straight up to the ceiling, out towards the point of impact. It was going out to a fulcrum point, to the end of a tide. It was a fluid mechanism driven out there by an automobile accident.

The fluid mechanism got out there and then stayed hung out there, because there was still a forward drive behind it. I guess you could call it a "limbo" injury. A limbo energy field was created. Why? I don't know—it just was. So the fluid mechanism and energy field got out there, and then I got a fulcrum point underneath him. I'm a living body, and I had a pair of hands underneath him, providing a fulcrum. He didn't express this condition until I put my hands underneath him, but as soon as I did put my hands there, as a living body, there was a focal point from which this limbo energy could spring.

So during the treatment, off this limbo energy went, and it stayed up there until whatever was necessary to neutralize it canceled it out, and then back it came again. Now the energy field was neutral. My fulcrum point was neutral before it started, and my fulcrum point was neutral after. But my fulcrum always is alive—it's a living fulcrum—so it was able to cancel the limbo energy field out. Now he doesn't have that pattern anymore. That answers the question about what is safe to take in. It is safe as long as you consider the fact that all that is taking place is an interchange of energy that came out of limbo and is going back to the same place.

Another point is that I didn't get exhausted by this process of treating him. No patient ever drains me. Yes, a patient can drain you. Somebody who's extremely weak, or someone who is a taker, can literally suck you dry, or someone who has too much energy can flood you. But nobody ever drains or floods me because I tune into my own inner Self, that part of me that's interchanging with the cerebrospinal fluid. When I begin a treatment, I contact my inner Self first; then I contact the patient's. Having these contacts, I say to their inner Boss, "Now you just do your own work, and leave me alone." Then there's no way they can touch me. But I've got to contact mine first and then the patient's.

In other words, in the treatment process, we're going to utilize that which automatically belongs to us. There is no need to think about giving or taking anything. We're back to basics. I've had young doctors in my office that literally were drained by patients of mine—I get all kinds of strange people as patients. It can be a real problem when you are dealing with people. So, yes, with the provisions I've described, I'll take anybody's problem into me.

Question: Because it has no place to stick?

There is no place for it to stop. It's just there for review and for me to experience what it takes to resolve as much as I can for that particular day.

All the corrections in any form of treatment always take place after you do the work. Nothing ever happens while you're there at the time you give a treatment. Occasionally, once or twice in two years, you might get someone that incidentally makes the correction while you're working on them. Most of the time it takes place between treatments. During the treatment, a change is simply initiated, and when the treatment is over, the patient is still arguing with their own Boss. They're arguing as they go out the door and all the way home.

Question: Would you treat, analyze the whole body no matter what the problem is?

I'm just going to meet whatever needs there are on that particular day. I'm not going to pick on them from one end to the other in every treatment. No. I'll just work on whatever needs to be done. This approach works because, even if you're picking on one little ring finger, you're picking on the whole body. I tune in on everything they own when I'm working, no matter where I'm working.

You have to get over the idea that the problem is the body. Forget about the body—it's just the baggage somebody came in with and parked on the table. Forget about it. The body is not the point—that's just the complaint department. That's just the ego there. That's why everybody wants to get well. That's what everybody exercises for. That's great. But it's still nothing more than a bag full of effects that's reacting to everything that's going on. This issue bothered me for a while. Why am I, as a physician, just taking care of a bunch of ego trips?

Well, unfortunately, that's what the world is—a bunch of ego trips. Therefore, somebody has got to take care of them, and why not take care of them efficiently?

If I am working with the ego-trip body purely to keep it amused, and to get it to a state of so-called physiologic health, that's very interesting. That's all people come in for. But I can also reach through the particular pattern of that body, not only to find Health, but also to find and arouse the inherent Mind of that individual and give it a little shot in the arm. Then perhaps that patient would get the hint and arouse their own internal capacity for human spiritual development. I never mention the word "spiritual" to them, and I have never mentioned it before to any other group. I have found you don't use that word, because it has connotations. But for me, when I work with my patients, I am purely interested in arousing the deepest level of their total awareness, whatever you call it. In this process, I'm teasing at something that's buried wherever they have buried it. I don't know where it's buried, I don't even ask, and I don't care. I just tease at it anyway. Meanwhile, more superficially, I'm seeking the layer that relates to healthy function for the problem that they came in with.

I'm absolutely not saying that I am giving a spiritual treatment. I don't want to be known as a spiritual healer. I'm not in the business of healing spiritually. However, my internalized goal is that I'm trying to touch the innermost part of the patient's being every single time I give a treatment. I've got a perfect excuse. They came to me for help, and I spell Help with a capital "H."

I strongly believe that the human body is the lowest form of energy we work with. But even though it's the lowest form, I'm thoroughly convinced that the human body has the intelligence to know what it needs to do to be well. It's constantly trying to improve its state. So we carry a base pattern of cellular function that exists for each individual cell which says, "The way I am is great, but I know I am tuned into something bigger, and I could be even better if I had a chance." Cells have a no-name intelligence that they are automatically functioning with. This is the only reason the body works. Otherwise, we'd be replacing a part every 15 minutes. Also, this is the only reason we can work with this approach. Any time we run into a block, a strain, or anything else that louses up the flow in any given area, we can just work around there until finally something happens which allows it to reestablish the flow. The cells only know one thing—which way is better. And that's the way they're going to go. I'm convinced of that.

I'm also convinced of the fact that if you take anybody and work with their mechanism purely at this fundamental level, they will achieve a result. In other words, if I only treat the strain to get rid of the problem, that's one level of treatment. If I treat it to get rid of the problem and at the same time tune into the whole mechanism, I'm going to get another result. If I treat the area with the idea of forgetting the fact that it's got a problem and literally try to bring the health out of it, to wake it up and say, "Hey, you're the one that's supposed to be doing the work here," and then tune that into the rest of the health pattern, and then tune that into the Boss that wants to take it upstairs, I will get another result. So you've got different levels of results depending upon the approach that you, as a physician, make.

We are programmed to think in terms of problems, and that is all we think about—we forget to go through that to the next layer. You can focus on getting rid of a strain in a hip, but you can also tune it into the rest of the leg. That's a better investment than the first approach. Then how about just forgetting about the problem? Where's the real health that would like to be there? Let's feel that flow move back through there, and let's hook it up to an even greater source. What I'm trying to say is that we stimulate from the lowest level to the highest level—we stimulate the whole chain. We're not treating just the body. If you're aware of that when you're working on this person, you're treating them from the foundation to the dome.

≈ ≈ ≈

It's the Boss that's doing the work. The physician tunes into his own Boss, and the physician tunes into the Boss of the patient. This is not a mechanical treatment.

Question: I'm wondering if there's any need or extra benefit from the patient trying to be conscious of the process of change?

No, it's not necessary. This mechanism is more than self-sustaining; it's literally self-creating. Things that are in constant motion don't require any attention. No, it's not necessary during the treatment.

⁀ ⁀ ⁀

Although if you have a patient who is so inclined, he can treat himself very easily. Every time he goes to bed at night, he can tune into his Boss and very quietly say to it, "Look, why don't you get rid of some more of this junk and allow me to move up the good part that's lying on the bottom?" Try asking to get rid of this bad stuff so the good stuff can come out.

Question: Is the progress a patient makes maintained?

It tends to spontaneously keep on going unless somebody gets hold of his head and runs him into a wall. In the beginning, the strain pattern is still there and is a little slippery, and if he gets an injury, it might cause the pattern to reoccur, but it would not necessarily reoccur with the same intensity, nor would it last as long, and it could be corrected more easily the second time around.

Responsibility of the Physician

Question: You once talked about the responsibility we have for our patients. You said it isn't our concern how or why the patient got to us and that we are not responsible for curing them. You said our only responsibility is to do the best we can at that moment. Can you talk more about this?

This was taught to me by one of my mentors, Dr. Charles, who practiced in Pontiac, Michigan. I had moved there in the middle of the Depression, 1936–37, and had gotten an office. There were 13 osteopaths in town at the time, and each of them sent me one case. They were being real "nice" to the young doctor who had just come to town, giving him some business–except that each case they sent me, either the guy was known never to pay his bill or he was going through town and was there for just one visit.

But Dr. Charles, with whom I later became acquainted in a very warm friendship and who became one of my mentors, sent me 100 of the finest patients he had in his practice the first year I was there. And he did so in such a way that I didn't know he was sending them. When I finally found out where they came from, I thanked him for it. He said to me, "You don't have to thank me. Patients don't belong to any doctor, although some doctors like to think they do." Doctors work behind closed doors. They say, "This is my patient, and you can't have him." But Dr. Charles believed patients should always go to doctors with a choice. They should always go to a hospital with a choice. They should always go anywhere with a choice, because 50% of the battle is when they accept the services from the physician they are going to. And he said, "Besides, if you hadn't taken care of them, they would have been right back," and he was right.

I've had a lot of patients who were just flat unhappy with me and sought other services. That's great, it's fine. I've got a lot of patients whom I truly wish would find somebody else to take care of them because our chemistries don't mix; they just rub me the wrong way. They're a drag. I'm not in sympathy with them. But I'm the only one in Dallas who uses this type of treatment I give, so I don't have a large choice. I can't send them anywhere else. But patients have the total freedom to be what they are. For better or worse, as a physician, you tend to attract whatever patients you are going to be responsible for. Sometimes you'll wish that whoever was in charge of allotting some of the strange ones would find some other doctor to take care of them.

⌐ ⌐ ⌐

Patients will not always respond the way I want them to, but that is not my responsibility. I am responsible to the "I-ness" that makes them that individual. I am not responsible to any of the "i" that makes them an ego. I am responsible to the capital "I" that makes them what they are. I am not responsible for the little "i" that makes up their name, denomination, sex, creed, color, or anything else. I can work with the capital "I" to the best of my ability on any given day, while the little "i" is functioning on whatever level, doing its thing. That's where my responsibility stops—that's the bottom line.

With anything that's initiated, their capital "I" is going to continue to work. It's liberated, free, and I can dismiss that case from my mind. I don't take my cases home with me mentally. Sometimes a patient comes to me in the morning, and they're as sick as can be. They think they should come back again that afternoon. But if I have listened to my inner "I" and listened to their inner "I" and have achieved something that feels like it's going to work, I don't have to worry about them. I'll tell them that I'll see them at their next regularly scheduled appointment. Something tells me I can forget about them. I don't go home and worry about them.

Each tissue has its own built-in time frame for healing. It takes 12 weeks for torn muscles or a broken bone to heal. In trauma, healing will take place within the context of and according to the anatomico-physiological nature of the tissue. It is a living process. If I accept that these are the ground rules and agree to listen to what those tissues are doing at any given stage, then I'm free simply to participate and share my responsibility for the time the patient is there, and then I'm done. I don't have to take them home. At the end of a day, I've worked hard, and I'm tired. But I don't have to worry or think about any of my patients.

It is my responsibility to give patients instructions when they leave the office if there's something they are supposed to do to supplement the care that I've started. But if they refuse to do it, that's their problem. I'm not going to worry about it. It is a pure frustration. It's rare that any patient assumes responsibility for themselves at any time, in any place, under any circumstance. I can generalize that statement and apply it to all people. Very few people will ever truly assume responsibility under any circumstance.

Question: But that doesn't mean that you can't help them?

You can still help them. But that is why I don't bother to tune into their superficial being, asking for their assistance. I tune in to the thing that will encourage them to help themselves anyway. If I didn't tune into that, I'd feel guilty for every treatment I gave. If they want to listen to themselves a little more closely, they can figure it out. Sometimes they'll actually do things without realizing why. Sometimes they'll go home and take a nap for an hour instead of rushing out to another appointment, doing this, that, and the other.

People in general have imprints of trauma and disease on many levels overlapping each other, which express a tremendous thickness that they can't get through in order to be themselves, or in order to take responsibility for their lives. To the extent that you're able to contact and awaken their own Silent Partner and begin to stimulate the dissolution of these overlapping patterns of inefficiency, you are really helping the person, and whether they know it or not is not the point. Who cares? All those layers of tensions want to go back to where they're pure limbo energy. These tensions fundamentally have nothing to do with the person. These tensions have assumed this pattern of injury, and now the person continues to carry it as a habit pattern, without even being aware that it is a habit pattern.

It's an easy subject to talk about, but it is one rough road to try to live, for the reason that each individual is primarily responsible for his own work to be done. There's no way I can make you do what I think you're supposed to do to get to where I think you ought to go. I couldn't force you if I put you under lock and key and force-fed you for the rest of your life—nothing is going to happen.

☙ ☙ ☙

I don't worry about whether a patient likes me or doesn't like me. If they don't like me, then they can find somebody they do like, and the patient will get well faster than they would have by hanging around my place. I've given money back to patients several times. They come in after three or four visits and say, "I think that you're doing nothing, and I'm not getting anywhere." They have so much pent-up frustration. I then respond, "Well, how many visits have you had, Mr. Smith?" He says, "This is the fourth treatment." Then I say, "Okay, here's a check for the other three visits, and there's no charge today, and I would like for you to find another physician." They usually then go out of the office sputtering and swearing, but they can't complain. And they can always call back six weeks or six months later and come on in. I've had some patients do this, and they can end up being the nicest patients you ever had in your life.

In the case where a patient is honestly disturbed by my treatment approach–this doesn't happen but once in three years–I don't hesitate to encourage them to go elsewhere. I'll pay them back.

The Potential for Results

I treated one woman for 18 months, and as it turned out, I had misdiagnosed the situation and couldn't really have helped her. She had accumulated a pretty good bill. I told her husband, "I'm sorry, I was on the wrong track the whole time. There's nothing I could have done even if I'd known about it, so let me write you a check for the year and a half's work." He replied, "No, things were at least a little bit more comfortable." She had a very severe form of tic douloureux, which was actually organic and could not respond to any type of functional treatment. There was no way she would ever get better–it was irreversible. He said, "No, if you want to write it for about half of it, I'll take that."

But, don't ever make the mistake of reaching a quick prognosis and calling something irreversible. If a patient walks into the office and they can say "hello," I know they're alive. I've tangled with dozens and dozens of problems that I knew full well, according to the books, you were not supposed to be able to do much with. But when we included a few little extra factors, and followed the patterns of motion and the things Dr. Still talked about, it was amazing how many loads of debris were washed off those problems and how finally the patients were able to make physiological changes.

One case like that was my friend with the shattered leg, whose legs remained ice cold months after the bony injuries had healed. This problem resolved when I found and treated an area of shock in the lumbar enlargement of the spinal cord. I've had several cases where one segment of the spinal cord is shocked. You can also see a shock in the thorax or some other part of the body.

There is a shock that comes with a myocardial infarction in which there is an implosion that literally shocks the whole chest. It's in a total state of shock, and you can feel it, if you develop your sense of touch. To treat it, you have to get into that thoracic area where all the cardiac autonomics are and wait until that shock dissipates. And it can dissipate just like that. All of a sudden you can feel it wash out of the chest. What is it? I don't know, and who cares? But this is what I mean by the potential that is there for those cases that from your medical training you *know* you can't help. There is some potential if you can find anything in a person which says, "I've got some vitality; now you figure out where to punch a hole in me, and I'll let some of this junk out, and then we'll see what I can do." If there's any potential at all, go ahead and work on them.

I treated a doctor who had severe back pain for 15 years, since being shot down in World War II. It took about three years to get his back to the point where the fibrosis he had come in with finally absorbed enough to let him be comfortable. I didn't see him for ten years, and then the problem kicked up again. His spinal cord had begun to deteriorate. He had gotten some sclerosis in his spinal cord, and so he came back in and has now regained 80% of his function and is doing great. There was a lot of irreversibility in that problem, but in spite of that, 30 years later, he still has gotten regeneration, which is pretty good. I had thought the best he could do was to hold things where they were and keep them from getting worse. But surprisingly, he restored about 80% of his function. He needs to have at least one treatment a month to maintain his gain, because that burned-out spinal cord has lost its insulation and has a tendency to drain out its energy. The cellular structure just can't hold a charge.

You won't always get all the results you want. I never have been satisfied with all the results I got with anybody, including the dramatic "cures." But at least you get the satisfaction of knowing that maybe that patient got the doors open for some more of that life and motion—that life in motion.

The Silent Partner

Question: Can you talk about what you call the "Silent Partner"?

Well, if I talk about it, that isn't what it is. One can only say that the pure "I" that represents me is my Silent Partner. It is the same Silent Partner as yours, the same Silent Partner that is in this room, and the same Silent Partner the insect I saw walking around has. It's all the same Silent Partner, and accepting and surrendering to it has to become a conscious experience. The Silent Partner is not anthropomorphic—it is itself. It has to be made a conscious awareness or knowing, but just the second you've got something that you can put your mental, intellectual finger on, that isn't it. But still it is something that is.

The Silent Partner can deliberately be appealed to or contacted on a one-on-one basis. Why and how it works, I don't know, and if I did know, that wouldn't be it. It's easier to demonstrate than it is to talk about. Right now I'm going to contact mine, and while keeping an awareness of mine, I'll contact yours. Now, I'm going to quit. If I contact yours and then quit contacting yours, I haven't changed it one way or the other. But it's more than an ordinary contact. Can you feel the difference? It is instant communication. And all that you are aware of is not it.

Through its transmutation, it has aroused an electrical potential, and I am aware of the system working in your body. I am not aware of the exact details, but I am aware of something going on within you because it has been activated. By what? The only source of power there is—the *Cause*. I contact the Cause first. Why do I contact the Cause first? Because I also am Cause. If you are going to be a patient of mine, and I would like to work with you in the most efficient way that I can for the short period of time you're going to be with me, then why not play with the Boss instead of playing with the secretary?

When you have contacted a patient in this way, you have not taken on the responsibility for that person with that contact. You are simply trying to say to that individual, "Look, Boss, you're already Boss in that area, and I know that when you do your work, you're going to do it just exactly the way you want it done. Now I would like you to wake up and do that work, although I'm not going to sit here and watch you do it." I approach it this way, because your Boss is far more knowledge-able and efficient than I am for whatever problems you've come to me for. I've aroused its antennae, and I'm asking it to go to work. But I'm not going to dictate how it's going to do its work, and it isn't up to me to sit there and watch it or concentrate on it. The quicker you can get away from it and just go back to pure surrender, the better.

All right, let's take this one step further. I'll contact my Silent Partner, then I'll contact yours, and then I'm going to surrender to it. Something happened didn't it? There's a difference. All of a sudden, you have the same process working for you, and I've lost my respon-sibility for it. It's going to be working, and now it's my job to get in there and do what I've got to do. See? You can talk about it, but there's nothing to talk about.

One thing you have to get over is the idea of relating to problems. Just like when we said the body isn't the point, it's also the case that disease is not the point. If you relate to problems, or you think about things in terms of problems, then all you've got are problems. All you have is one effect on top of another effect on top of another effect. You never get to the cause. So forget about problems.

The Silent Partner *is,* and that's all there is to it. So why not call it into action? When you get to talking about how to use it, I have given you the simplest answer that there is to give, and I haven't any more idea when I'm contacting mine what I'm contacting than I know about the man in the moon. Because if I did know, then it wouldn't be a Silent Partner. That would be making it part of the same limited-effect world that everything else our mind can touch is. I'm contacting it and surrendering to it—it's as simple as that. If you make it any more complicated, you're dead—nothing's happening. That's all there is to it. That's what A.T. Still is talking about when he says, "God, of the mind the nature." That's what he is referring to.

Question: So it seems like part of our job is to open to that, to surrender to God?

Actually it boils down to what do you surrender to now? Your Silent Partner is a fulcrum point; it's absolutely still. There's no energy in motion in the Silent Partner, none. It's all energy, but it's not in motion. Actually it is the source of energy, the state from which energy comes. It isn't energy in motion, it's just pure potency. It's omnipotent. There is no motion, and yet it's all motion. It just is, and you surrender to it. Feel the stillness that has developed in this room. It's the same stillness. Can you feel it? It's all the same stillness, and you can feel it, but it's not something that you work at. If you work at it, you're missing it. It's a living stillness that our conscious awareness can be aware of. This conscious awareness is with our big Mind, not our little mind. Awareness is the acceptance of something.

While this may sound esoteric, it is a tangible experience. Once in a while when I'm treating patients in my office, you can take the stillness in that room, cut it with a knife, and make an igloo out of it—it gets that quiet. What brings it on? I haven't any idea, and who cares? It is there to meet the need for something that is going on for that particular individual. Where it comes from and where it disappears to is not important. It's a way of life, a way of Life with a capital

"L." So that's what it is. Don't make it complicated. You can contact your own Silent Partner right now, and you can contact someone else's and then surrender to theirs. Everybody can do it; we all have the same resources.

It is possible to learn to live in the "presence," as Joel Goldsmith calls it, 24 hours a day. But, we're always forgetting this, being distracted by this world we're walking around in. But it's possible, in spite of the fact we're walking through this world, always to be in constant surrender to this thing you just made contact with. It's simply a matter of continuing to surrender as a conscious awareness experience, and it gets to be a habit. It is practically impossible for us to do this always because we're human beings and live in this world. I get tired, and while I'm driving home, someone cuts me off and I get mad. So it's hard to do it, but it's as simple as that—a conscious, personal, even super-personal surrender to this stillness that's part of our being.

Attainment

Question: Ultimately is there an attainment of some sort?

Well, you can think of the attainment in terms of a habit. This way of being really becomes a habit. Moment by moment, you attune to the stillness and reattune to it and reattune to it. And there's no point in time where it just happens—you just go along and that's the way it is—because this is something dynamic. This dynamic is intrinsic in it, and it is constantly in motion—or nonmotion. So there's no way that you can just plug in and go. It is always a conscious effort. It's part of the individual's responsibility to continually maintain his plug in that place.

This is true for all personal growth. Any spiritual individual of whom we know has made and sustained this contact. Walt Whitman had it. What do you think he wrote his *Leaves of Grass* from? When he was writing, he was tuned into this thing. Dr. Sutherland had it when he was developing his cranial concept. Dr. Still worked for 15 solid years on seeking this thing and discovering what constitutes a new program for treating people.

In any major creative expression, in artists or anyone else, this is where they get their creative instincts from. They are tuned into it, perhaps not as a conscious effort, but they are tuned into it nonetheless. Because if someone wants to create that Sistine Chapel ceiling, they say, "I've got to have all the help I can get." They're automatically tuning into and using it. But how many people in the world are literally going to make the effort to use it? There are very few people who try to make it a continuous surrendering process. It takes practice and experience. It took those people years and years to create some of the things they did. They didn't get it overnight.

It's important to remember that in every instance it is the process of attunement that is the point. The attainment, and the result it brings, is not something you should ever be concerned with. It is about attunement, not attainment. Beyond the attunement itself, everything else that takes place is simply a matter of expression; it is manifestation. This is a case of "effects" again, and if you get hung up in that as attainment, then you have crossed your wires and you are back into the state of egotism.

Joel Goldsmith, author of *The Mystical I,* brings out a very good point along these lines. He says that if you can actually live continuously in that awareness, in complete surrender, you automatically find that there is some peace and contentment. The same problems that would have driven you crazy, you just go ahead and take care of.

I get absolutely no satisfaction in achieving a cure in a very difficult case. It is no gratification to me to see somebody respond to the treatment I've been giving them for six months, and all of a sudden, a 20-year experience has been wiped out, and they're back to a state of health. There's no gratification or contentment in it for me—not one bit. People may say, "Isn't it wonderful? Look what you did for Mr. Smith. He can play golf and make another million dollars, and before that, he was in bed for six solid months. Doesn't it give you a real glow of satisfaction?" No, none. I could not care less. There is no gratification at all, none. You think I'm kidding. But that was Mr. Smith's responsibility in the first place, and what about the other five difficult cases I've got in my practice? Why aren't they responding the same way? I can't use the same answers for them. So I'm still stuck with the responsibility of finding out how do I surrender so that this creative thing can be transmuted for the next one.

Besides, Mr. Smith's particular circumstances, and all the things it took to be the problems that he was, were his individual problems and had nothing to do with my care. I just happened to be the lever, the fulcrum, a still point. And a still point has no name, it has no ego, it has nothing. It's motionless, and yet it is all potency, and the potency that he utilized for his particular problem came out of a still point from my Silent Partner and his Silent Partner. They get the credit for whatever happened. So why be gratified?

I'm very grateful for the fact that he has made this tremendous change. But I am grateful for his sake, not for mine. I take no credit for any of it—it doesn't belong to me. I am grateful as can be, and I've surrendered to his total new health pattern, to his own internal being, so it can keep him that way.

I love my work and am grateful for the opportunity to do it. It doesn't ultimately have anything to do with anybody else, but it's a wonderful thing to have the opportunity to be reminded to contact your Silent Partner, and to surrender again and again. This opportunity is what all the cases I see represent, and it's a good thing.

If I were to get gratification from a case, that emotion arises from my ego, my little-"m" mind. Then my intellectual mind begins to analyze, saying, "Let's see, now I did such and so at that particular time and got this kind of result." You end up analyzing everything that took place which possibly contributed to why he did this or that. But at the root, in the background, his anatomicophysiological structure is nothing more that a mass of cells that are going into flexion/external rotation and extension/internal rotation ten times a minute, and they're doing all the hard work. You're kind of teasing them once in a while, and there's no way you'll ever be able to analyze how it happened. It's all past history anyway. Now he's a new man, and this is a new day, and we're supposed to be living in the now. So why get emotionally satisfied over something that's already been accomplished? What's the next goal for that man?

Also, if you get emotionally satisfied or gratified by what you succeed in, then you also create for yourself the unfortunate position of being frustrated, disappointed, and unhappy when you don't succeed. You set up a block of energy that you're going to have to fight. Ultimately, you don't make it happen when it is good, and you also don't make it not happen when it isn't.

Goals

You asked me, What's the goal? You can't really think about it in terms of seeking something. People have a tendency in their spiritual work to think, "If I live right, I'm going to get a mansion over there on the sunny side of heaven." It's a goal—if I do the things I'm supposed to do, then something good will happen. Well, who writes the goals? If I could tune in to my Silent Partner, practice the presence, and literally be all the things that I've been talking about all the years of my life—if I could reach a point of such attunement—then my creative energy would keep going on and doing its thing. When there aren't any ego trips involved, people are responding in whatever way to the work that I'm doing, and something is happening. When I get through with this piece of work, am I supposed to punch in on the clock and say, "Here, now I have a goal"? Goals have to disappear with everything else.

You do experience some sense of comfort. You experience the ability to surrender into your work, to surrender into a total interchange in which you're sharing something in which everything happens, and you don't have to put a label on it. There's no idea that: "I got satisfaction out of that. I'm contented because this is going on. There's peace in my world because...." That kind of thinking doesn't make sense to me. What are you doing this for? How long is it going to be at peace? The next job's going to demand more work. It is a state of conscious balanced interchange. If one could actually do it, there would be no time to do anything except just to be comfortably doing what you're doing without thinking about the word "comfort."

We all need, in the beginning, something to get hold of. There is a structure to the treatment. But in the end, there really is nothing to hold onto. There is a goal, but it's a goal in which it isn't important that it is or is not.

The practice of medicine is a humbling experience. You get humble when you've got a case and you're banging up against the wall. So many of these patients have made the rounds, have gone through any number of clinics, and now they stumble into your office, saying, "I've been told I'd better see you. Mrs. So-and-so said how much you'd helped her." Then you realize what a monster you have got here.

Lots of patients come in with problems, and nobody really knows what's going on. Some patients will overstate their problem and others will understate it. But if you tune in to your Silent Partner and to theirs in preparation to even talk to them, you can smell the problems. You can feel the layers of crud and other things 40 feet deep. That tends to be a humbling experience. The only trouble is, if you get real proud of being humble, then automatically you have got a whole other set of blocks to go through—so forget it. Your job is just to get in there and start pitching bricks to find out where the problem is, because most of them are covered up with so much rubble, they've forgotten where they are buried. You just have to start throwing off the bricks.

In your practice, 99.9% of what you see is ordinary stuff that makes you say to yourself, "Why do I have to take care of this?" It's the little complaint: "I've got a twist in my little finger"; "My neck is sore"; "My little girl has a tonsil that looks a little red." This is the kind of ordinary stuff that makes up your practice, and you get lazy, saying, "Let's take a quick look at that. Now, good-bye." But with this type of work, you're going to prove to yourself that you can't afford to be lazy. You've got to tune into your Silent Partner, surrender to it, and surrender to theirs. Give it that little extra attention. Maybe it will take a couple of minutes to really look at it, to really see it, to really hear what they're trying to say about it.

What are you doing? You are not being a psychologist. However, automatically you're discharging whatever is there. You are discharging some of the crud that's permitting the problem to be there. You're giving a service from the inside out, even when the complaint is a minor one. And it takes a lot of work to do it on an hour-after-hour basis. It takes a lot of conscious effort for a while, until it gets to be a habit. No, it isn't really a habit—it's just that you get to a point where it takes less to remind yourself to do it.

In the average practice, there isn't that much going on to get excited about, even in mine—and I probably draw more strange cases than anybody in the city. I think it's just as important that we be as responsible for that minor case that walks in the office as the one that really excites our interest. But it is hard work to do it continuously, and there are hard days in which it feels like it's almost impossible to do it. Everyone has their ups and downs. Don't get me wrong, though— any type of practice is a lot of fun because there are so many types of people it keeps you entertained.

What we're talking about here isn't exclusive to the world of doctors. It's the same rules as anywhere else. I had an engineer friend in Michigan who had 30 engineers in his organization. He had a heart attack, and I used to go out to the house to treat him. Upon reflecting on his business, he realized he had three engineers who were really great. He could drop dead, and his business could go on just as well as it ever did. Then there was a bunch of engineers in the middle that were good. And at the bottom, he always seemed to have three that were just no good. The point is, if you're going to play the game and be in the top 10%, you have to use all your ability to function; it simply takes more to do it. And I don't care what game it's in.

We, as doctors, spend four years getting a piece of paper that looks beautiful and hangs on the wall. Then we are free to practice egoism and make a million dollars: "That's Dr. Brown in his new fast car." Very satisfying? Very dull to me—I care less than nothing for that. I used medical school and that piece of paper that I got as an excuse to allow me to practice the way I choose to practice. The deal of being a physician, or any other honored profession, is that it is literally just an avenue for work. That's all it is.

Here is a funny case that's worth talking about because it shows you how ridiculous being a physician is. When I was practicing in Michigan, this young man came into my office, and he had deeply fibrotic bilateral psoasitis. He couldn't straighten up and had lots of pain. I practically had to carry him onto the table, and then his knees would be sticking way up in the air. That was back in the days when I was working harder; I wasn't doing what I am doing now. I worked on that guy, Joe, three times a week for two and a half months, and at the end of that time, when he came into the office and lay down on the table, he looked just the same. He said he had to leave town, so we parted company. I was glad to get rid of him; I was getting tired of him.

Sometime later, a new patient came in and had arthritis and a dozen other complaints. He said that Joe had sent him up to see me and had told him I could fix him in one treatment. A few months later, another guy came in, and he had everything in the book, and he was only going to be in town for a week, but that's all right, because Joe told him he was going to be cured in one treatment. Finally, a year later, Joe came in, and he was a big, strapping guy and straight as a string. He said, "I'm telling you, I wasn't in Florida three weeks before I was straightened up, could do anything I wanted, had put on 50 pounds of weight, and I've never felt so great in my life. Have you been getting those people I've sent you?" I said, "Joe, do you remember how long it took to treat you?" "Yeah," he said, "you gave it to me in practically no time at all." "It may have been no time for you, but it was two and a half months of hard work for me!"

This shows that time is not time. Joe had no remembrance of how long it took. It went down the drain along with the energy that caused his problems.

Question: If we are students and the person we're working with is the teacher, how do we start learning? Do we start just by getting our hands on people, trying to tune in, and allow that to take us?

That's right, just be a student for the rest of your life. I've been a student for the past 35 years and a doctor for the first ten before that, and I haven't even gotten started yet.

Question: Are there any wrong alleys to go down once you start?

There are plenty of wrong alleys. The results you get will demonstrate that fact; you'll not always get the results you want. This will inform you that you have to shift gears. If I had treated just the leg of the man with the shattered femur, and I hadn't paid any attention to the spinal cord, I could have treated that leg for the next five years and might eventually have made it feel better, but I would have been working a long way away from the place that was giving the orders to that situation.

I had to know enough anatomy and physiology to go up to where the problem was getting its prime orders from, which was creating an effect down in the leg. In this case, one thing wasn't causing the other; it was all the same problem. I had to know enough anatomy and physiology to go to the centers that were going to have control over the peripheral tissue that needed influencing. You can play with the peripheral tissue—patients always want you to put your hands on the area they complain about—but that's just your point of reference. You need to go from that peripheral area to the point that's going to have more impact on it. Patients are going to complain about where it hurts, but in this case, the condition that's actually influencing that complaint is the total mechanism that it takes to be a leg.

If you get poor results, it can be because you may not have gotten to some of the more important centers or because the stupidity of the patient is such that when they go home, they screw up your treatment. This happens all the time, almost routinely. This isn't your problem. They don't eat right, this is their weekend for a binge, they got into another fight with their husband or wife, and so on. So they are spending their resources and wasting them in some other way, and they come back and the area is messed up again, although not as badly, in spite of what they do or don't do.

Teaching

You know it's very difficult to teach this type of work to somebody. A physician may come in and say, "Dr. Becker, I want to study with you until I can begin to understand what's going on here." But the first thing I've had to do with these people, and it is a very rare one that will do it, is to tell them, "The first person that's going to have to make a change is you. Anything that you've ever learned before in your life, forget it." I tell them, "I have no answers here. You're not going to learn anything here, but when you get through, you'll be pointed in a direction to go, and you'll have to find it out the hard way yourself. But you're going to have to drop everything—drop your identity, drop your 'Doctor'—and just start off with a clean slate when you step up to the table to find out."

As I said, it is the rare physician-student who is willing to do this. I end up struggling with their personalities, their egos. Whenever I would let them have their hands on a patient I was working with, I would feel them trying to project their energy into the situation, trying to pick up something of what was going on. Interestingly enough, patients would get overtreated in this way. Patients would comment on it—they felt an overload.

When you're dealing with the highest known energy that's available, it doesn't want anybody interfering with what it's trying to do. It reacts when somebody is monitoring it with an intellectual analyzer. I gave up letting students have their hands on the patient while I was treating.

I also never let the physician-student talk to me when I'm treating a patient. If you want to know about this patient, ask me before they come in or after they leave. I won't let the student even open their mouth to say this is a woman or a man when the patient is in this office. I do this because if you say anything about that patient, such as this little area of strain is thus and so, the patient immediately forms 27 diagnoses and goes home and tells their families and friends about all the magnificent things that are wrong with them, and then you've got to overcome that.

It's hard work to teach somebody to do this work. You can teach them that this is what you would like them to lean towards. You can teach them that this is the way that perhaps they can start working out for themselves what they want to do with it. But you can't learn this work by studying me or anyone else doing it. It's literally a self-taught process.

This work is a flowing thing. You've got to learn to flow from one patient to the next, and it's not the type of flow that perhaps you're thinking about. Every patient who walks in the office has got their own flow according to their own level of operation. So you've got to tune in to where they are at, so that you can know what you're going to do with what they have. Then when you leave them, they have still got to be flowing in their own way, but better than when they came. This means that it's an individualized treatment each time that patient comes into the office. If you ever have to give the same treatment twice, you screwed up the last one. You didn't do anything. Things may not be much different at the next visit, but something should be happening with every treatment.

The biggest problem we have amongst those who do this work, which is the hardest thing to accept as physicians, is that the patient walking into your office is alive. This is true even amongst those who studied under William G. Sutherland. Despite his hounding, Dr. Sutherland could get very few of us to realize that we were dealing with a living anatomic body that is smarter than we are. It's alive! It's awake! It lives and says, "You can come and pick on me. I'll do anything you want me to, even let you create problems with me, as we try and get back my health." But no matter how you say it to physician-students, they say, "Yeah, yeah, I know, but where was the lesion?"

⤳ ⤳ ⤳

A few years ago, there was a conference, and I was assigned the job of arranging things for this guest speaker who had an hour-long time slot to give a lecture, demonstrate his technique, and have everybody go to the tables and practice. Five minutes before he was to start, I was told he wasn't coming. I now had an hour that had to be occupied by something, because you don't go to one of our conferences to loaf around. Our group is probably one of the most devoted groups of physicians in the United States. When they go to a conference, they work hard. In fact, it's hard to chase them out of the conference area at the end of the day—they're so busy treating each other.

I scratched my head over how to fill the hour and then decided to have them make a physical examination without going through their usual routine of testing for motion. I told half of them to lie down on the tables, and I told the other half, "Start at the head, and just put your hands on the head, then come down to the neck, come down to the chest, go down each arm, go down through the abdomen and pelvis, and go all the way to the feet. Take 30 minutes and don't *do* a thing. Just sit there and feel what you can feel." I didn't say a thing about where to feel from or what to feel for. I just said, "Feel what you can feel. Sense what the physiologic motion of the patient is doing." They had 30 minutes to do this, and then they were to switch partners.

I spent the hour going around the room saying, "Cut it out! I didn't say *test* for motion; I said *feel* for motion." I just kept slapping them down so they simply had to sit there and just observe. It was a sight: Here were 50 osteopaths with busy practices, used to chugging down the road, trying to sit still for 30 minutes. The interesting thing was that in that simple exercise, as they got into the process of literally feeling with energy of their own, they became participators. They were practicing participatory quantum mechanics. They were arousing all the energies of the patients as well as their own. There was enough energy welling up out of that room that you could have made building blocks and built a house out of the stuff. It was amazing.

At least 25 of them came up to me later to say that this was the finest treatment they had ever had. It's interesting. It was a diagnosis session, but they all got treated. The other interesting thing was that it didn't arouse one bit of curiosity amongst them about how they could go home and do this. They were willing to experience it, but they weren't interested in taking the responsibility to develop it. But it was a very clear demonstration of the potential of this work. I was amazed to see how much energy 50 people could generate.

I have treated many dozens of physicians or their families with various problems, some very serious and chronic, through this type of service, which allows their physiologic function to do its own work. They come, get results, and they're not even curious when I get through. They don't even ask questions and never ask how they can use this in their practice. They just barely say thank you. What we do is a perfectly valid thing; there's nothing secretive about it. But apparently some people just aren't open enough to realize that. They need the protection of their closed political system. It wasn't that they thought they weren't capable of doing it. They just didn't make any statement at all.

But there was one physician who did, an M.D. who was shot down in World War II and had terrible back problems for about 15 years. He came to see me upon the urging of another doctor. I would work on him for about 15 minutes and then say, "See you next week at the same time." That was our total conversation for the next three months. He never said one word, and I just did what I was supposed to do. Then he'd go on his way. Three months later, he said, "Do you mind telling me something about this stuff?" I said, "Well, I was waiting for you to ask." We went to lunch and talked about it in detail for one and a half hours. He understood the basic principle perfectly—everything in the body wants to do what it wants to do and will do so if you just give it the chance. If allowed to do so, it's going to take any trauma and shorten and minimize the aftereffects of it. It's going to take any disease and run it through the whole cycle efficiently.

ON TREATMENT

The Restoration of Health

The purpose of the kind of care I give is strictly to allow your system to have *all* the resources that are available for it to work with. I treat anybody and anything. The questions I am primarily interested in are: Where are the resources being blocked? Where are the areas that need to be put back into action again? Could you handle this trouble more efficiently if your system were in tune? I pay far more attention to seeing that things are doing what they're supposed to be doing than I pay to what we call problems. I do not try to fix your problems; I am not interested in wiping your faces. I want to get underneath the crud and say to the part that is healthy, "Look, you are supposed to be up here doing this work."

In other words, I'm treating to restore health; I'm not treating to correct the problem. In treating this way, I have opened the doors for the body to try to do what it wants to with its own living forces.

Question: Why can't it do that without your help?

It can.

Question: But why doesn't it? You've described that one reason the body doesn't make a good or full recovery is that there are other compounding factors that the body is trying to pay attention to. What do you do with the other factors? Are they still there after your treatment?

That's right. But after the treatment, they're now being cleaned out by a better, more healthy mechanism than the one that was trying to do it before and that wasn't being very successful.

Question: How about trauma versus disease? Is there a difference in how you approach a mechanical ailment as opposed to a disease?

No. You are trying to separate mechanical problems from disease problems, but they cannot be separated. If the tissue is in strain—for example, a leg has an internal rotation strain—all the fascias and everything else are in a state of lowered resistance. If anything penetrated the skin, the fascias and the lymphatics would not drain the area as well as they should. It would become a local site for potential infections. But once things are back where they belong and functioning well, everything that leg needs is going out to it, and what needs clearing out is coming back. It's now in a healthy state. As Dr. Still said, if everything from foundation to dome is freely moving in its pattern, then every part of the body will be working in the way it's supposed to work, and physiologically, it's going to do the things it needs in order to handle anything that tries to get in. This freely moving mechanism helps conquer whatever is put in there.

To help anything, trauma or disease, you reach for the primary tissues in body physiology. You look to see if the autonomic nervous system—the sympathetics and parasympathetics—is in perfect balance. The autonomic nervous system controls the blood vessels, which in turn controls the interchange of fluids, which in turn controls other things. You ask yourself: Is the autonomic nervous system free to do what it wants to do? Is the drainage from the venous and the lymphatic systems in the areas of stress free to get out?

Question: Do you ever try to deal with mental illness?

Only from the standpoint that I try to restore the batteries of these people, which are usually down. When you have a patient in whom you don't feel the normal high-voltage pattern of health, if you can charge them up, they're going to do better.

Question: How about surgery?

It's absolutely essential for a lot of conditions. However, it is a traumatic thing, and sometimes, while it takes care of one problem, it creates another. The best definition I can think of is that surgery is organized trauma. There are a lot of things it's essential for, but it is still organized trauma.

I occasionally get a case I need to send to surgery. I get a lot of people who come in with what they call disk problems, although only one out of 20 of them really are. For those who really do have a disk problem that eventually requires surgery, the three-month treatment program I have them on to see if they really need surgery prepares all those tissues so that they are a lot better equipped to take it.

To have gotten a disk problem in the first place, you would have had to put a lot of strain on the other tissues as well. The disk is just one of the complaining tissues. There has been a total strain to the lower back, and in addition, the disk had a herniation. We have to wash that shock out of all those tissues. If you get the shock out of them, a lot of times, even if the disk is ruptured, it ceases to hurt, and they don't need to have surgery. On the other hand, if it's ruptured too much, it's going to put pressure on some nerve, and it's going to say that it can't take it anymore. If you take the shock out of all the connective tissues with preoperative treatment, the surgery will likely be a lot more successful, and the recovery will be a lot faster. Then postoperatively, it's the same thing—you've got to wash the shock of surgery out of them afterwards.

With surgery, it helps if it is done carefully by a surgeon who is going to get in there, do skillful work, and get out again. There are even a few individuals who are willing to say a prayer over you before they start cutting, although they get criticized for it. A while ago there was a picture in the *Medical World News* of a surgeon saying solemn words over a patient, and they quoted him as saying that medicine was now recognizing the fact that it pays to call on the Boss every once in a while. Nine months later, there are still letters to the editor howling about it, calling it the most unscientific thing they've ever heard of. On the contrary, I thought it was about time somebody admitted they did that.

Question: What happens to your body if you're surgically changed?

It adapts to it. Surgery is just organized trauma.

Rules for Treating

When you're dealing with the body's inherent forces, you've got to write a whole new set of rules for the game. In an ordinary practice, you can see a red throat, decide that the patient needs penicillin, and give it to him. That's an external view of the event. Or you can put a patient with psoasitis on a machine to stimulate the area with galvanic current and then put him in a whirlpool for 15 minutes. These are mechanical gadgets that you're directing, and that's fine. They work in the way they're supposed to work. On the other hand, you could get your hands on these patients and provide a focal point through which the local tissue changes can work themselves out. In the case of the psoasitis, those other modes of treatment are working on the voluntary muscular system that is cramping and complaining. But you can also contact an involuntary system that is working ten times a minute at pumping through that tight area.

It generally takes seven to ten minutes for some change to get started while your hands are on a patient. Just because your hands are there and you have tuned in to the patient doesn't mean that everything is going to immediately just happen. The body is designed to work deliberately. Long before we had automobiles, long before we even had wheels, man was walking around using the same equipment we are using today, and the body's response to a treatment takes time. It takes time to give a treatment, although it's rare that a case has to stay on my table for more than 20 minutes. But that's 20 long minutes, and how many shots of penicillin can I give in 20 minutes? That's the reason a lot of our profession has quit using any hands-on treatment, because they can see five patients in that same length of time.

But in this approach, you're dealing with the native resources of the human physiology, operating ten times a minute for x number of minutes, in order to achieve a point in which this total connective tissue mechanism and the total body of fluids—including cerebrospinal and lymphatic fluid—is interchanging with the Breath of Life. It sometimes takes seven to ten minutes for this mass of fluid and its enclosing membranes to slow down and go through a still point, during which this interchange takes place, and then all the orders flood out to release the spasm. The time frames are set by the mechanisms of the body; it takes longer to use this type of treatment because that's the way the body is designed. You can't get around it.

The characteristic of physiologic forces is that they will do their own thing if you tease them enough. Then when they finally get around to really making their corrections, they'll usually do it between treatments. Patients often don't feel like anything is happening, and then finally some big shift takes place. I've been through that so many times with so many people. But that's all right because I don't listen to the patient to assess progress. I tune in to what their body is reporting back, what changes it is trying to make, what is its relation to what was there before I started, and what goals does it have for the next few hours.

"Boosting" Treatment Results

You can try to affect the body with a galvanic current, and it will have an effect, but these mechanical gadgets are doing things from the outside. Unless you monitor the body, you don't know what effect it is having. Usually the physical therapist puts the patient on a machine, walks off, and comes back in 15 minutes to take them off it. Maybe for a few minutes it feels pretty good to that sick tissue. Then all of a sudden, you're asking the sick tissue to respond in a way that it can't, and it's getting tired out. If you had your hand on those tissues, you would know this.

I used to have a diathermy machine in the office; I had the idea that I would heat one patient up while I was working on somebody else. Then one day, I finally got smart and put my hands on those tissues to see what was happening. The first patient I checked, in three minutes there was a signal from the tissues, "Hey, this feels pretty good." After five minutes, that signal turned off and it started building up pressure. I had that patient there for 15 minutes. So I gave him five minutes of treatment and ten minutes of trauma. The next patient I put on the diathermy had two minutes of treatment and 13 minutes of trauma. The next patient took ten minutes to signal it had enough, leaving five minutes of trauma. I discovered that the tissues definitely respond to all these gadgets that we use, but your hands have to be there to monitor it to know when the change you are seeking has taken place. It turned out to be $350 wasted. I threw the machine away. Again, when we get to playing with the science of allowing physiologic function to do its own thing, you have got to obey the rules.

⇋ ⇋ ⇋

A few colleagues of mine are always trying to come up with ways of boosting up patients to try to have them temporarily have more energy present during a treatment. Their idea is that if they can do this, then more can be accomplished. But that isn't the way it works, because if you have tuned into your Boss and their Boss, the no-name body physiology is going to use only the specific amount of energy required for its use. With these boosting methods, you may feel like more is going on, but it's not.

You cannot force this work; it simply won't work. I can give a treatment to any one of you in this room, and by using direct action, the Boss, and all the energy and knowledge that I have, I can literally force any one of you to make the correction that I want six weeks from now. I can do it. I've done it. What takes place is that for six solid weeks you are totally miserable. You get all kinds of reactions, and I have to cool you off for six weeks while you make the changes I want to take place. I stir up all this nonsense and overload you; it just doesn't fit the gears. I don't do you any harm, but I don't like that position.

Types of Motion

At this point in the meeting, Dr. Becker read his paper, "Motion—The Key to Diagnosis and Treatment," which appears in Life in Motion.

The first type of motion I talked about in the article is gross voluntary movement. Muscles are designed to do things, to be used as they walk around and do their various duties. They are able to do these things because of the gross patterns of motion and movement available to them. So when you take hold of anybody, you're automatically in contact with these gross patterns. Patients are going to be hitching themselves around on the table, so you've got to include that gross voluntary movement in your treatments.

I worked on a little 18-month-old the other day, and she was bound and determined to move about. She took me all over that office trying to work on her. I got hold of her pelvis, and just followed her around the office. But all the while I was following the gross patterns of her movements, I was also reading the other patterns of movement, and all the while working until finally the correction took place.

The second type of motion I described in the article is the secondary respiratory movement. Every time you take a breath, everything in you, clear down to your feet, is moving. As you are working, you can include that in your awareness. The third pattern of movement I described is this fluctuation that's moving ten times a minute. If you can be subtle and just a little patient with yourself, you can feel this slight external and internal rotation of the bilateral structures and the flexion and extension of the midline structure. You can be aware of that motion or note the lack of it.

The Large Tide

Then there is this large tide-like motion. That's an interesting one that I first became aware of about ten years ago in some people I was treating. It's obviously always been there, but it was startling at first. I had been working for about 15 or 20 minutes on somebody, and all of a sudden, I was aware of the fact that it felt like the whole patient was expanding. It was like watching fingers of the tide coming in, seeping through the tissues. It did this four or five times. I just kept watching it, thinking, "This is fun; what's going on?" Finally, all of a sudden, something happened and the whole thing just melted out. Apparently, it went through one of those relative still points, and there wasn't any need for it to work again.

So where does this large tide come from? Does it come from the top, bottom, or sides? Is it inside and does it decide to come out? Does it start anywhere or quit anywhere? I haven't the foggiest idea. It could be a harmonic. There are lots of postulated explanations for the cerebrospinal fluid's ten-times-a-minute fluctuation. But it's easier to try to explain that tidal fluctuation, because that's a body of fluid within a certain amount of space. But with this large tide, I have no idea. All I know is that it demonstrates itself.

Question: Have you found it in everyone?

No, I have not. In fact, I don't even look for it. I have found that if you have somebody with a lot of general systemic problems—things involving the total body physiology—you might have it occur. If you have a patient that has either one fairly large area or enough smaller ones involved, then eventually, sometime during a treatment program, it probably will show up. Apparently, a patient has to have a fairly large interrelated volume of problems for it to come into action.

I actually think it's there all the time, but like anything else, if there is no problem, it's strictly in interchange with the total universe. If there is no problem, you just feel a simple rhythm. I think we're in simple rhythm with the farthest stars, ten times a minute by way of the cerebrospinal fluid and a minute and a half apart for this large tide. I think this large tide is always there, but when there's a resistance to it, as in a gross layered problem, we become aware of it. That's all I know about it, except that I am convinced that this large tide is a manifested form of one of our patterns of liquid function or living function that's supposed to be, and it's there for a purpose. It isn't there to create problems; it's there to solve problems.

Question: Is it something you work with by applying your treatment techniques?

I do. I use the whole fascial system. When I feel it start to come in, I just start going where it wants to go and act like a fulcrum to contain it. I don't impose any channels I want it to go in, but I give it a nice tight fit so it will keep going where there's work to do. I don't let it just dissipate blindly, but I give it room to play in. I'm strictly there to hold the stuff into a focus so the work can be accomplished.

Question: Is that why you use a fulcrum, to contain things?

That's one of the reasons a fulcrum is used.

In our patients, we are dealing with the combination of all of these motions. We're not using them individually or going through one stage after another. We're just taking them in combination. All these motions are going on simultaneously, and we're trying to interpret the total pattern that is demonstrating itself. We're making observations: What are these movements doing to the body as it lies there? What is this total pattern of movement doing to this area that we're trying to work on? How is it twisting that area, if there is a twist? Does it feel like it belongs to this, that, and the other?

Fulcrums

Question: Could you explain more about fulcrums?

A fulcrum is a still point, a source of power. Fulcrums aren't levers; fulcrums are still points. Out of the fulcrums flow the levers. The tissues that you've got a hold of are the levers that are going to be doing the moving around for you. They are the ones that are going to take the energy and do the twisting with it. They have available not only their own energy but also the energy they get from your fulcrum points. Automatically, they are taking advantage of your reference point, which in this case is a fulcrum—whether it's one hand, two hands, an elbow, a knee, or whatever you've got against them.

The fulcrum is the source of power. It's the point of reference from which the levers of your body—as a floating, palpating person—plus the levers of the patient's body are trying to struggle with the problem. Having established a fulcrum point with some part of your body, you are operating through levers, while at the same time, their body is providing levers. In this system, your fulcrum point is a neutral point for the staging of the struggle or fight that needs to take place.

Question: So you're centering it too?

I don't know that you're centering it. All I know is that you give them an arena in which they can do their thing. There's no way to say that you're centering anything. I don't know what's going to happen. It may center and it may not. It may go more peripheral or it may go more central. You just provide the battleground.

Question: I see.

No, you don't see and you never will. I haven't seen it yet, but I don't worry about that.

≈ ≈ ≈

You can't describe function. I can't describe or tell you how it works. I know the rules. I know the principle: If I move my arm from one point to another, I have to work from a fulcrum point. Otherwise, I couldn't do it. I have to move from back in my body somewhere; I have to move from a fulcrum point. Therefore, I'm providing a fulcrum point for the patient, who has a no-name body physiology, to have something happen from within themselves. I don't understand how it does it, and I couldn't care less. But I do know the principle. I've got to have the point from which it can happen. There's always a fulcrum for any change.

When I work on someone's hip the way I was showing you, I rest my elbows on my thighs. This gives me points of reference. I am a physician, I want to get something done in a reasonable period of time, and I am not going to sit there for 24 hours wondering what is going on. I want to know when to start and when to quit working with the patient. For this, you have to have a point of reference. This allows you and the patient to cooperate efficiently for that day's treatment, and it helps to get the treatment done within a reasonable time frame.

You could accomplish the same thing by sitting there and telling the patient to pick up his leg and do this or that with it. But how long are you going to take to treat that person? An hour later, you still don't know if you've found his release point—you haven't any reference point. You're the physician. This is the reason you're there. You are there because you've broken out of the standard political system and accepted the fact that your no-name body physiology and the patient's no-name body physiology are smarter than you are. So you agree to take these two intelligent pieces, put them together, and let things happen. But you've got to have some kind of contact to know what is really going on.

If I lift my elbows and don't have any other support for my arms, I still have a fulcrum, but now my fulcrum is my whole body. It makes it much harder to know exactly what's going on if you're sitting out here at the end of the lever. Remember, in this work, we're not talking about a gross test for motion; we're talking about a microscopic test for motion, a millimeter at the most. You've got to work with a short leverage.

You sense through the fulcrum. The sense of touch comes from the sensory area of the brain to the hand, but you are feeling from you. You sense through the fulcrum with your Oneness—the Boss. The Boss is in the fulcrum. A simple iron bar under a rock that has a fulcrum is the same thing as the God that's centering you. A fulcrum is a fulcrum. It's a source of power.

You contact your stillness, you contact the patient's stillness, and from that time on, you're feeling. That's all there is to it. But you're not a passive machine. Put your hands under that cup you are holding and register that it is a cup. Now contact your stillness, contact the stillness of that cup, and all of a sudden, it's a different cup. All of a sudden, you've got a different feel of it. That's because there's a stillness between every pair of levers and between atoms.

You cannot describe function. You can describe the end results of function, but there's no way that you can define the function itself. You can describe the things that are doing the function, but the function is not describable. But you don't have to worry about it because it's already taking place anyway. If it needs help, you just establish a fulcrum, establish a point from which function can take off and do its thing. This takes a lot of strain off you. You don't have to make the gastric juices dissolve the sandwich eaten today. The body physiology is going to do it—you just encourage the process.

Palpatory Skills

You're going to develop your palpatory skills a lot faster than I did. It took four solid years, from 1945 to 1949, for my stupid palpatory sensory cells to wake up and feel the things that I was supposed to be picking up. Our sense of touch is absolutely dead, except to say, "Here's a cup of coffee," or something like that. You've been using your eyes since you were born. You haven't used them with the skill of an artist, but you've always been seeing. You've always been hearing, although not with the skill of a musician. To awaken the sense of touch to be as sensitive as your eyes or your ears is truly a development that takes time. It takes at least a year or two.

The more people you get your hands on, the more strange things you'll feel and the less you'll understand them. Even so, you're constantly improving your sense of touch. Finally, there comes a time when, because you know your anatomy and physiology, you can analyze and say this is probably the reason this patient is having this particular complaint. You can decide that this particular area probably needs attention because it feels a little bit like if I can just break open the stuff that's going on in there and let it dissipate, probably something would happen. Although, there's no sure thing; it may not happen. But at least your sense of touch has given you a clue as to where to look. It takes some time to develop a sense of touch. I don't care if you have full knowledge of what a fulcrum is and know all the answers about it, you still would have to take a long time to develop the sense of touch. You're dealing with the finite body and its own lack of development. There's no rush. I've only been doing it consciously on every patient I've seen for the last 35 years, and I'm still developing it.

Your sense of touch has to be projected from up in your brain. As an exercise, lay your hand on the person sitting next to you. Put your hand on their shoulder or whatever part you want. Then, just sit there a minute, observing the breath, exhaling and inhaling a couple of times. Now, without moving your hand, project your sense of touch from your brain down to your hand. Sense from your fingers, from your whole hand up to your brain for about 30 seconds. Now turn on your own Silent Partner. Sense from your brain down to your hand. Now tune in on their Silent Partner and continue to sense from your brain to your hand. Now back off and just go back to the first level of contact you made. It's like turning a rheostat from level to level. These are your tools.

I think it's also important that you realize that your palpatory skills are quantum mechanical skills. There's no way you can be an independent observer. Whenever you lay your hands on anybody, automatically you have started modifying whatever they are. It doesn't make a bit of difference what the problem is, you have modified them. The mere fact that you have made an examination means that you have already started something for that body to try to help itself. Quantum mechanics is a sharing experience. That's all it means.[5]

Patterns of Motion in Treatment

The various types of motion I've described, together with your palpatory skills, are the primary tools in both diagnosis and treatment. In the treatment phase, they are part of the treatment principles. You're playing with all these movements in each one of the treatment principles we usually describe—exaggeration, direct action, disengagement, and opposing physiologic motion.

For example, if I strain a finger joint in external rotation, I can exaggerate it and find the point at which it became an external rotation strain. I can tease it and exaggerate it until I find that exact point. It feels neutral—I don't feel anything. The joint hurts when it's carried back the other way, but if I carry it to the point where it went into strain, it doesn't hurt a bit. It is strictly neutral. So I can support it right there and allow these four major movements which are going on all the time to work on it, and they tease those ligaments and eventually make a correction there. Then this joint mechanism comes back and is in neutral again, without strain.

You can accomplish the same thing with direct action. You can carry the affected part back towards the point at which it should be—although in an acute case, the patient won't like this. You find the point somewhere in between where it is and back towards where you'd like for it to be again. You find the point at which it's neutral again. It's all just balanced fulcrum points; you've always got to look for those things. You just work to keep neutralizing it until you get it to a point where you feel, "Ah, there it is." Then just hold that balance

---

5. Dr. Becker uses the term "quantum mechanical skills" in a way alluded to in a *Science News* article (May 22, 1976): "Thus quantum mechanics makes the observer a participator. Not only in Heisenberg's sense that the observer disturbs what he measures, but in the more profound sense that his choices of what to measure will determine what he finds. Reality has no objective existence apart from the act of observation."

until it goes through a treatment cycle. It will argue, twist, and turn, and then it'll release. It will correct itself. Disengagement is usually used to help get a strain, or mechanism, to a point where it can exaggerate or go into direct action.

Use of Compression

Often in my treatments, I apply a little compression at the start. My understanding is that a person is centered somewhere—there is a hub. To aid in the treatment process, I can apply a controlled compression towards that center from wherever I am on any strain pattern. This is a controlled compression; I don't just shove it back in there. Again, I am functioning as a participator, a participator in quantum mechanics. If I first apply a little compression towards the center and then add in the exaggeration, direct action, or whatever I want, I find I get results a lot faster and get a better correction.

The compression is going towards the point out of which energy comes. The energy that is manifesting is radiating further and further out to the end of the limb. If I compress towards the point from which the power comes, I'm taking it back towards its built-in fulcrum point. So I, myself, use compression in practically every treatment I give. I use a modified form of compression plus exaggeration, direct action, opposing physiologic motion, or what have you, depending on what the tissues are trying to do.

In working on a particular area, it can take five or six minutes to finally get to the point where, using compression and this, that, and the other, I find the exact point of neutral. Even then, I can continue to refine it. Once you find that neutral point, you want to support it. It's neutral. My hands are fulcrum points, and they're quiet. I've applied some energy from my fulcrum points into the body's resources, resources that have been going on all the time I've been finding the point. The body is going through its ten-times-a-minute motion anyway, and I just cooperate with it, and now it's going to work for me. As it goes to work, I've discovered that it's automatically going into exaggeration or opposing physiologic motion or whatever because the body's mechanism knows just exactly what it took to produce the strain, and it's going to go through the same thing getting out.

It's not going to go into these patterns of movement because I started it, but because that is the way it works. It's applying its own principles, and all of a sudden, it releases and there it goes. It goes through a quiet period, and then you can just feel the four major fluid movements that we talked about. They just feel like big waves. Then I can go back and test the joint motion. It flows in external rotation, it flows in internal rotation. The joint feels like it's supposed to feel. The no-name body physiology uses the same principles to do its own work that we incorporate as physicians.

Diagnosis

We all have our own unique patterns. None of us is symmetrical. My pelvis, for example, is twisted so my neutral stance is a little askew. Because of this, everything on the right side of my body should naturally be in external rotation, and everything on the left side is supposed to be in internal rotation. If I come to you complaining of my right leg and you find it goes more freely into internal rotation, while the rest of that side of the body goes more freely into external rotation, then you have found that I've created an internal rotation strain. It's something that has gone against the grain of my normal mechanics. One day I rode in a boat and produced just exactly that problem.

I was riding across a very choppy lake and got thoroughly chilled. I braced my leg in internal rotation to keep from getting tossed out of the boat, and this put the whole leg into an internal rotation strain pattern. When I finally figured this out, I realized this pattern didn't fit me and walking around with it was making me tired. It put a drag on my muscles and everything else. I had gone to some of my colleagues, but they had not been able to help. So I finally figured it out myself and started teasing on it. Eventually, I found the point of balance for it, gave it some support, and after a while, it felt as if that whole leg was going to come off. If you looked at it, it wasn't actually doing anything, but it felt like it was trying to come up this way and that. It was bucking that boat all the way across the lake until it suddenly shifted gears, relaxed, and moved back into external rotation. It treated itself.

≈ ≈ ≈

When the occiput is low on one side, it means that all the dense fascias that fasten to the base of the skull are going to reflect this. There are 34 muscles fastened to the base of the skull, 17 on one side and 17 on the other. In addition to those muscles, there are fascias starting at the base of the skull which are continuous down to the feet. When the occiput is low on one side, that side of the occiput is in relative external rotation, and you'll find that everything associated with it on that side is in relative external rotation and everything on the other side is in relative internal rotation. You might have a little scoliosis in the body associated with this.

When the sacrum goes down on one side, there's also a little curvature. But as long as that curvature can wiggle freely, it doesn't make any difference how many curves there are. As long as the spine is going into its inherent flexion-extension movements freely, there's no problem. It's when you break that pattern that there's trouble. For example, when you get a normally externally rotated rib that all of a sudden becomes an internally rotated rib, then you've got a rib dysfunction, and that will really hurt. It doesn't fit the pattern anymore. You get hold of that rib cage and discover the patient has been leaning over and has twisted the ribs the wrong way. Then you figure out some way to get hold of that thing so that it releases and gets back to its relative external rotation position again. The pain will go away; they'll lose their "pleurisy" in a hurry.

There are all kinds of patterns in the cranium itself, and here again, as long as it is freely rocking back and forth the way it's designed to, you have no particular symptoms. But if it's restricted—if you have a blow, whiplash injury, trauma, or anything that locks this thing and holds it in a given pattern and does not let it go through its full range of motion—then you're interfering with function. You're affecting the tug and pull of the dura, which can interfere with the venous drainage and the cerebrospinal fluid absorption, resulting in relative congestion of the central nervous system. Then you can have all kinds of symptoms. You can have symptoms from the 12 pairs of cranial nerves, including the vagus nerve, which has actions all the way down to the large intestine. So there are a wide variety of symptoms you can have due to modifications of a complicated mechanism.

Locked Sacrum

The Tide has a nourishing, trophic effect on the body. Think about it for a minute: The cerebrospinal fluid fluctuates 100 times in ten minutes. What has this done? Ten times a minute every cell in the body has been massaged—every cell up and down that whole spine, including the spinal cord, muscles, and everything else.

I had a patient who had locked up his sacrum in an accident 25 years ago, and his upper back muscles felt just like glass. His body hadn't gotten a good massaging for 25 years. As you might expect, given the age of the trauma, it took some time to restore health. It took nine months, not to *correct* the sacrum to be right again, but to restore it to normal function. It took nine months to dissolve enough mass of the glue, fibrous tissue, and what have you. I kept encouraging it, and finally, he came in and his sacrum was rocking like it was supposed to between the pelvic bones. Some time before that he had already lost all the symptoms that were bothering him, but I just kept playing with it until it got to doing what it wanted to. Finally, and physiologically, his no-name body reported: "Okay, I'm back on the beam. Now why don't you leave me alone?" So I fired him. He came back eight years later for a relatively minor complaint, and I found the muscles of that whole upper thoracic area were just as good as new. They had completely healed themselves from eight years of being massaged.

You can see the importance of reading what the no-name, physiological functioning would like to be doing in any given patient if it could be an unencumbered no-name body. Think about how many potentials there are for helping anybody. The person doesn't even have to have a complaint. All you need is a universal no-name body physiology that says: "I have rules for my health, and those rules are being compromised." And if the rules are being compromised, you can go after the situation.

At least 35% of all automobile accident cases still hang on to a locked mechanism. It doesn't make any difference whether they're hit from the side, front, or back, as long as they're hit.

Question: Is this indefinite unless you correct it?

Yes, although fortunately for most people, they adapt to it, and they don't really hurt that bad. In fact, when you discover the locked mechanism, you often have to remind them that they had an accident. The ten-times-a-minute fluctuation is still going on, but it is doing so poorly and less efficiently.

∽ ∽ ∽

The sacrum is a wedge-shaped mechanism lying between the pelvic bones. In the thorax, we're aware of the fact that the scapulae, sternum, and ribs are all separate features with some degree of independent mobility—in the same way that the sacrum and two pelvic bones should have some degree of independent function. With trauma, the sacrum can get glued or locked in between the two pelvic bones, and then they function as one piece. For instance, in an automobile accident, you're thrown away from the seat, and then you come slamming back down. This can lock the involuntary motion of the sacrum.

To diagnose a locked sacrum, you can put one hand under the sacrum, cupping it so your fingertips are up near the base. With the other arm, bridge the two ilia to monitor their movement. Then have the patient dorsiflex his ankles and then extend them—have the patient move his ankles up and down, up and down, and observe if the sacrum is free to move between the pelvic bones. If it is free, you will feel the pelvis move as three independent pieces. If it is not, the sacrum and the ilia are going to be carried up together, and they're going to be carried down together as one piece. If the two pelvic bones and the sacrum are moving independently of each other, it is not a locked sacrum. The sacrum may not be doing all it's supposed to be doing, but at least it's not locked.

When monitoring the sacrum, don't push up on it with your hand. Instead, lean a little bit onto your elbow, which then can function as a fulcrum point. Lean just a little bit; don't lean on that fulcrum point so much as to make it lock. That fulcrum point has to be able to move; otherwise the structure you're contacting can't move. It's a floating fulcrum point. It's a very little motion. We're not talking about walking across the room; we're talking about a few millimeters.

By altering the pressure on your elbow, you can change the depth of your sensing. By putting on more pressure, automatically you'll sense more deeply into the sacrum. If you use less pressure, you'll get a more shallow sense. In other words, as I'm leaning here onto my elbow, I get deeper and deeper and deeper, and the lighter on my elbow I get, the more shallow I get. As I get firmer and firmer and firmer, with my hand under the sacrum, I can feel and be in direct contact with the psoas muscles.

Clinical Conditions

Question: What is your experience with phantom limb pain?

I never had one get better. They hurt just as bad after I've treated them as they did before. There are a lot of situations that are irreversible. Of course, I only think it's irreversible because I haven't figured out how to make it work in the several cases I have had.

Question: Epilepsy?

I've treated a number of cases of people with epilepsy who were taking ten doses of anticonvulsants a day. After they got some treatment over a period of time, they were way overmedicated, and finally we had to cut them down to two or three in order to accomplish the same thing. My idea of what happened is that because of the treatment and its effects on the autonomics and the orders that go towards digestion of food, the patient was finally able to absorb and utilize all that medicine. So all of a sudden, those patients were actually receiving ten doses a day and had to be cut back.

Treating a Frozen Shoulder

You're all going to see cases of frozen shoulder in your life. I had a lady nine years ago who had bilateral frozen shoulders. She could get her arm up just so far, and then she'd pass out on me. She had bilateral brachial neuritis, and this had been going on for many years. She'd been trying all kinds of treatment for a long time before I ever saw her, and when she came to me, I worked on her with every technique that was ever invented. I tried everything in the book to get those shoulders to let loose.   The shoulder is quite a structure. The only place where the upper extremity hangs onto your bony skeleton is at the medial end of the clavicle as it joins into the sternum. It is the only bony contact the arm has with the rest of the body. Everything else is a suspensory mechanism of ligaments, tendons, and fascias extending up the neck, over the thorax, and down to the hip. Everything else is hanging in space.

At the end of three months of treatment, this woman's shoulders were a little more comfortable, but as far as getting her arm to move more, we weren't getting anywhere. Then one day she was lying on the table and I took my shoe off and put my foot up in her axilla. I used my palpatory sense of touch right through the bottom of my foot, trying to feel what was going on. With that, a thought occurred to me, and simultaneously she reported that what I was doing felt good. I wasn't putting very much pressure up into her axilla, and I thought to myself, "You've created a fulcrum point, how about putting a crutch there?" I did just that and it helped her.

To use this method, adjust the crutch at the right height to go with whatever shoes the patient generally wears. It is adjusted to fit so it just exactly reaches the top of the axilla. Then the only thing they do is to use the handles to steer the crutches as they walk on them. They don't lean on them at all; they just walk normally with the crutch under the arm. They use it with every single step they take from the time they're on their feet in the morning until they go to bed at night. The crutch is a fulcrum point, and with every single step, they stretch, rest, stretch, rest, and stretch all the tissue involved. Then don't have them come back for three months. This is what I had that woman do, and when she came back, her shoulders were fine.

I've used the crutch method on over 200 people since, and if they're willing to walk and follow the exercise, they can walk it off. It's so simple, it works. The reason it works is that you have established a fulcrum point. You have this ten-times-a-minute mechanism working away on the inside, and you're giving it a fulcrum point to work over.

If the patient insists on coming into the office for a treatment, then all I do is to take my shoe off and put my foot up in the axilla, support it, test it out, see how it's coming along, and tell him to get out and walk some more. Some of them take longer than three months to get better, and some of them take less. But it's rare that I've ever had one come back and say, "I'm exactly the same as I was." There are only two people who came back and said they couldn't tolerate the crutch. One of them, I don't know why; the other had undergone a massive breast operation, and she was just too sensitive up in there.

The only time I've seen patients have any trouble with this approach is when they try to change shoes and the height of the crutch ends up being wrong. Either they have to reach to get over the crutch or they have to hunker down to get to it. In these cases, they're no longer physiologically in balance. Then it's just a question of making it the right height again. The biggest problem I've had is with the medical supply place where patients go to get the crutches. The patients are always being told that they are using the crutches the wrong way and that the crutches are the wrong height. Because of this, I usually have the patients come back to the office, and I adjust the crutch to get it just right for them.

It doesn't matter how they use the crutch, whether they take the crutch with the step or whether they go counter step, as long as they just steer it with the handle. It makes no difference how they do it, as long as they're getting a little passive push, pull, push, pull movement in that shoulder girdle sometime during that step.

If you ever get any frozen shoulder cases in your office, you'll discover why I like that trick. I flatly refuse to treat them anymore; I have never learned anything that does the job like the crutch does.

Patients will get relief. Some will stay with it just to a point, and they'll still have a certain amount of limited motion, but the shoulder is so free by comparison, they just get tired of fooling around with the crutch and don't follow through. If they really have a red-hot problem, it will be two to three weeks before they'll see any relief. There's an awful lot going on in that shoulder area. Remember the anatomical pictures of all that is in the axilla? Well that's how much stuff has to be given a bath. There's a lot of material that requires attention in there, and it's not going to respond just because you told it to. This process is not one of mind over matter. It's a matter of explaining it to the mind.

2. USING THE STILLNESS

This is an edited transcription of a tape-recorded correspondence from Dr. Becker to his close colleague, Anne L. Wales, D.O., in the early 1970's.

ANNE, THIS MORNING I want to discuss the use of stillness in a treatment program. We have previously talked about how I applied it to myself and was able to obtain results for two chronic problems. Now, I would like to discuss with you the use of it in the treatment of any case that walks into the office. I am trying to bring into focus a way of thinking, a way of being, and a way of using the stillness objectively and subjectively in the diagnosis and treatment of our cases.

Stillness, to me, is the very key to what Dr. Will [Sutherland] was trying to give us. In his various lectures, we came down to a still point. He made statements like, "allow physiologic function to manifest its own unerring potency rather than use blind force from without."[1] A.T. Still wrote in his *Autobiography* [p. 148] what I think is the true definition of osteopathy: "I hope all who may read after my pen will see that I am fully convinced that God, of the mind of nature, has proven His ability to plan (if plan be necessary) and to make or furnish laws of self, without patterns, for the myriads of forms of animated beings; and to thoroughly equip them for the duties of life, with their engines and batteries of motor force all in action."

───────

1. "...that fundamental principle advocated in cranial technic, viz: allowing the physiological function within to manifest its unerring potency, rather than the application of blind force from without" (Preface to the Reprint Edition. W.G. Sutherland, *The Cranial Bowl*, 1947).

Let's go next to an article I read by an eastern philosopher who was discussing the mystery of time [*Main Currents of Modern Thought*, Sept./ Oct. 1970]. He said that both space and time are two aspects of the most fundamental quality of life—movement. And based on direct experience, the Buddha stressed the dynamic character of reality, contrasting this to the generally prevailing notion of that time of a static atmaveda in which an eternal and unchangeable entity was proclaimed. The author said that, in fact, the original concept of "atman" was that of a "universal rhythmic force, the living breath of life," comparable to the Greek "pneumatos" [spirit] which pervaded the individual as well as the universe.[2]

He is talking about the reality of a dynamic, direct experience that is this stillness. It isn't what we call the still point—there are trillions of those. It is this stillness. It is stillness which is the motive force in the concept I use in my clinical practice. I definitely utilize the stillness as the motive force for securing changes in the patients.

I discovered a very beautiful description of the stillness written by another eastern philosopher. This man was listening to an artist playing a very complicated Indian musical instrument. The musician was playing beautifully, his hands were rippling across the strings, he was getting the right tone quality as a result of the right tensity on the strings and as a result of his plucking them correctly. The listener goes on to write:

> A strange thing was going on in the space which is the mind. It had been watching the graceful movements of the fingers, listening to the sweet sounds, observing the nodding heads and the rhythmical hands of the silent people. Suddenly the watcher, the listener, disappeared; he had not been lulled into abeyance by the melodious strings, but was totally absent. There was only the vast space which is the mind. All the things of the earth and of man were in it, but they were at the extreme outer edges, dim and far off. Within the space where nothing was, there

---

2. Atman: the Self; spirit; eternal principle present in the heart of every living being.

was a movement, and the movement was stillness. It was a deep, vast movement, without direction, without motive, which began from the outer edges, and with incredible strength was coming towards the center—a center that is everywhere within the stillness, within the motion which is space. This center is total aloneness, uncontaminated, unknowable, a solitude which is not isolation, which has no end and no beginning. It is complete in itself, and not made; the outer edges are in it but not of it. It is there, but not within the scope of man's mind. It is the whole, the totality, but not approachable.[3]

This certainly takes us back to some of the things that Will used to talk about—liquid light, the sheet lightning in the cloud, the invisible energies that create the X-ray image. It is the clinical experience of utilizing this stillness, this total energy, this total body, this total force, in the concept of the treatment program that I wish to talk about briefly this morning.

A patient comes in with any given problem, and when I get through with the history—get through with the conversation that's necessary to get them onto the table—I get my hands under the given area of problem and I try to be aware of stillness. Not a still point, but a stillness that is that individual. You can only be conscious of stillness, you cannot palpate stillness with your hands. The stillness is that which centers every molecule of being of that living body. The body physiology is the outward expression of that stillness. They are in total unity, in balanced interchange. In health, it is a free-flowing interchange. In disease and in trauma, patterns of disability are set up that have the stillness within them. So, the energy from that motive power is built into these patterns of disability as it is into the health.

The patterns of disability are present because of all the factors it took to produce them—the twists, the strains, the endotoxin, the what have you. They are present, and they too are subject to the

---

3. J. Krishnamurti, *Commentaries on Living*, 3rd series.

motive power of the stillness. Body physiology does not choose to allow that body to continue in ill health or in trauma. It chooses to correct that problem back towards free interchange and function with stillness—a state which we call health.

So when I get my hands on this patient, I establish a palpable contact of thinking, feeling, knowing fingers. I take hold of that problem with a knowledge of the body physiology of that part of the body—a total synthesis of understanding including its ligamentous-articular mechanism, its fluid dynamics, its interchange of lymphatics, its arterial flow of blood and venous drainage. The total picture from our training gives a dynamic understanding of what I am palpating, what is there in my hands. As soon as I am aware of stillness as the motive power that is in command of this case, then my hands begin to palpate and feel the shift of the elements of body physiology and their response to this motive power coming from the stillness. It is more that just a sense of motion. It's a living entity of interchange that is taking place. It is a true physiological picturing of the pattern of body physiology as it exists in its present problem as brought to the office.

My hands are sensing the total pattern of the disease process, the traumatic process—all the elements of total body physiology that are manifesting as the traumatic or disease process of function within this system. My hands—my thinking, feeling, knowing fingers—can feel the outward manifestations of life as time and space and movement in this existing problem within the patient. This is palpable to the hands and to the sensorium. It can also be observed in the way the patient walks and can be heard in the way the patient describes the story to the physician. It's the sensory experience of the effects of this problem upon the patient, and all this is available to the sensorium of the physician.

We have discussed two points so far. One is the awareness or consciousness of stillness, and this is a product of mind. This is the use of mind. This is the ability to realize, to know, to experience the stillness, and this has to come through awareness and consciousness of mind. The second point is that this working mechanism is palpable to the trained touch of thinking, seeing, feeling, knowing fingers. It is possible to feel the manifestations of change that are taking place in the tissues as motivated by the stillness that is the patient. When we become aware or conscious of it doing its work within the patient, here is where we have a law of physiologic function within to manifest its own unerring potency. Let's rephrase that a little by saying, allowing physiologic function within to manifest as the result of potency or stillness in action within this patient.

I, as a physician, am deeply conscious that I am sharing the experience, through my thinking, feeling, knowing fingers, of the motions, mobility, and functions that are taking place within the disease and traumatic conditions of this patient. Through the synthesis of my knowledge of anatomy and physiology and as I sense the totality of body physiology at work within that patient, I am consciously experiencing and am aware of sharing the experience of this traumatic or disease process within the body physiology. Because of my knowledge of anatomy and physiology and its functioning in the body, I am able to sense this function taking place while the motive power of stillness is releasing into action.

Now the treatment process of utilizing stillness becomes simple. One attempts to understand and feel the interchange, the rhythmic interchange, the total interchange between the stillness. The stillness is that which we are consciously aware of in the centering of the total being of the body that we are working with. We are conscious of this total stillness within this patient. We are aware of the stillness. We can feel mentally, mind-wise, consciousness-wise, awareness-wise. We know that we have this stillness. We are very definitely aware of it.

With our hands upon this problem that's deep within our patient, whether it's a traumatic or disease process, we can palpate with our hands the interchange that is taking place between the universal, dynamic, alive stillness and the disease or traumatic problem that we are working with. We can feel this palpating with thinking, feeling, knowing fingers. We can palpate the interchange between the stillness and problem. And when we can sense this interchange actively taking place between the stillness and the problem—when we sense that the body physiology has become part of and is sharing stillness in the problem and with the problem, and is interchanging with it to dissipate the traumatic and disease process that is in the body—we know that our treatment program is through for that day, for that is all that the body physiology needs. It is a permissive thing. As much of that problem as is possible for that given day will begin to dissipate back into the stillness.

Let us make a brief comparison here. We have our stillness, which motivates all that is and which is the source of all energy for all body physiology. We have a body physiology interchanging with stillness in health. Place your hands under any healthy area of the patient and be aware of stillness. Feel the body physiology of the healthy part of the body in free interchange with stillness. Palpate the total interchange of the forces of energy flowing from stillness. It's a question of sensing the fact that there is an interchange between stillness and health. There is as much energy flowing into body physiology as there is flowing back to be dissipated into stillness. There is a total interchange, an ebb and flow. With your hands on a healthy part of the body, you can feel this interchange of stillness and health within the body as a free interchange and total dissipation in both directions. There is no problem—it's freedom. With your hands under a problem, you share the experience as a physician, you share the experience of the problem in the patient. You experience the stillness with its motivating energy centering the total body. You can sense the interchange between stillness and the problem. You can feel the shifting dynamics of function of the body physiology as it relates to the problem within itself and as it attempts to become free again in its total interchange with stillness. This is the simplicity of sensing body physiological function releasing and dissipating congestive forces, tensions, tensities, ligamentous-articular strains, and toxic effects. This is the sense of the total organization of body physiology working with and being motivated by the energy of stillness to create a pattern of change, a pattern of correction. In this way, it is a treatment program in which health is related to a return to the freedom of interchange between body physiology and stillness.

Well, I probably haven't expressed it too well, Anne. But, I feel very strongly that we have the opportunity to go deeper into the study of stillness. I believe we have the conscious right as physicians to make this stillness a living part of our dynamics in the diagnosis, in the treatment program, and in the care of health for our patients. I told you before about my experience of utilizing it as self-treatment. In that particular case, I did not attempt to palpate the changes taking place within my body physiology because I was the subjective subject being treated, and I could experience through my sensorium the changes taking place in body physiology. My awareness was mind awareness, mind consciousness of stillness. My body's physiological responses to this treatment program for myself were sensorially felt through my subjective senses of body physiology.

In my application of this to a patient, my mind awareness is on the totality of stillness that is the patient's total self while my hands are palpating. My thinking, feeling, knowing fingers can feel, know, experience, and share with the body physiology of the patient the dynamics of the interchange between the problem within the patient and the awareness of stillness in the patient, which I hold in my mind. When I sense this interchange taking place through my hands as a palpable mechanism and through my mind as an awareness of the stillness interchanging with body physiology, then the treatment is complete. The challenge in my treatment program is to recognize the point at which I know that this interchange is taking place, to recognize the end of that particular treatment. All that will take place in a treatment on a particular day is determined by the permissiveness of the body's physiological process—the time, tensity, degree, and period of disability that is present in the patient. The problem is going to respond in its total capacity in relationship to all the factors it took to produce it. And it is going to respond to the point of permissiveness for that particular day and that particular treatment. And so my challenge is to recognize when this interchange between stillness and body physiology has reached this point of interchange, and then I can let go for that particular day. Enough, I'll talk to you again, Anne.

3. A Concept for Health, Trauma, and Disease

and

Rhythmic Balanced Interchange Technique

This paper was written by Dr. Becker as a summary of his own understanding and approach to treatment. He wrote it for his own use and never sought to have it published, although he did share it with colleagues. The paper was first written in 1972, and then was revised in May 1974 and January 1975. This is the 1975 version.

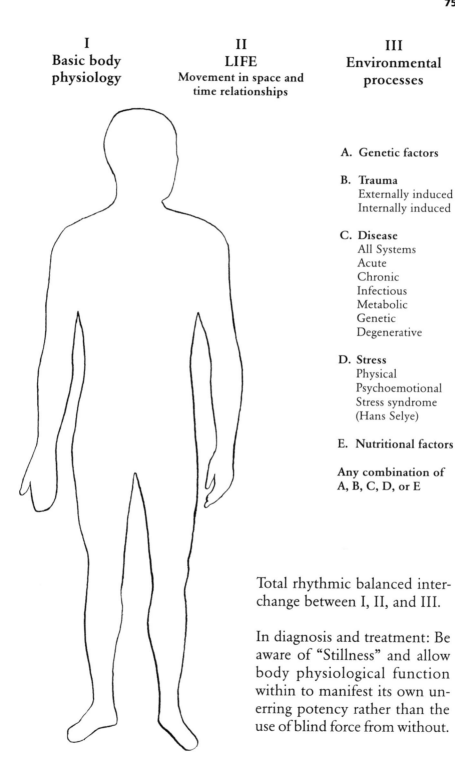

I
Basic body physiology

II
LIFE
Movement in space and
time relationships

III
Environmental processes

A. Genetic factors

B. **Trauma**
   Externally induced
   Internally induced

C. **Disease**
   All Systems
   Acute
   Chronic
   Infectious
   Metabolic
   Genetic
   Degenerative

D. **Stress**
   Physical
   Psychoemotional
   Stress syndrome
   (Hans Selye)

E. **Nutritional factors**

**Any combination of
A, B, C, D, or E**

Total rhythmic balanced interchange between I, II, and III.

In diagnosis and treatment: Be aware of "Stillness" and allow body physiological function within to manifest its own unerring potency rather than the use of blind force from without.

A CONCEPT FOR HEALTH, TRAUMA, AND DISEASE

BODY PHYSIOLOGY DEMONSTRATES THE following principles:
    1. LIFE is
    2. manifested through space and time as movement
    3. to demonstrate as body physiological function.

Life cannot be defined. It can be described. Time, space, and movement are the manifestations of life, from its highest spiritual manifestations down to the simplest physical phenomena. Life includes Stillness and space/time :: movement to demonstrate as body physiological function.[1]

Health: Body physiological functioning (anatomicophysiological mobility, motility, fluid balanced interchange) (space/time :: movement) and the Stillness (potency) of life manifest total freedom in rhythmic balanced interchange.

Trauma, disease, et cetera: Body physiological functioning (anatomicophysiological mobility, motility, fluid balanced interchange) (space/time :: movement) and the Stillness (potency) of life manifest limited rhythmic balanced interchange specific for each trauma, disease, or other limited entity.

The Stillness of life is directly experienced as a dynamic character of reality through awareness (consciousness). Space/time :: movement of body physiological functioning is directly experienced as a dynamic character of reality through awareness (consciousness) and the physical senses, including palpation.

The use of this knowledge can be described in several ways.

To evaluate body physiological functioning, it is necessary to be aware of Stillness through knowing consciousness of this dynamic factor of life and at the same time to be aware of space/time :: movement

---

1. The mathematical symbol "::" indicates "proportion"—a proportional relationship between parts. In a letter to a colleague, Dr. Becker quoted an author he had read as saying that both space and time are two aspects of the most fundamental quality of life—movement.

in body physiological functioning through the physical senses, including palpation. The Stillness of life and the space/time :: movement of body physiological functioning of life are inseparable although differing in their functioning capacities. They are dynamically in rhythmic balanced interchange.

Life can be accurately evaluated through awareness (consciousness) for the factor of Stillness (potency) and through awareness (consciousness) and the physical senses, including palpation, for the space/time :: movement of the body physiological functioning.

To be aware of Stillness and Know (Be Still and Know) for the Stillness factor of life is to actively and dynamically function with the space/time :: movement factors of body physiological functioning of life, which is sensed through awareness and the physical senses, including palpation.

In clinical application, be aware of the Stillness of life through awareness (consciousness) *and* of body physiological functioning of life through awareness and the physical senses, including palpation. Utilize the energies of the Stillness (potency) and those of body physiological functioning in their own dynamically rhythmic balanced interchange for diagnosis and treatment in health, trauma, and disease.

To state it more simply: Be aware (conscious) of Stillness (potency) and allow body physiological functioning to manifest its own unerring potency rather than the use of blind force from without.

RHYTHMIC BALANCED INTERCHANGE TECHNIQUES

Techniques to Achieve Balance in Physiological Functioning in Anatomicophysiological Mechanisms

Rhythmic balanced interchange techniques are a direct one-on-one application of the resources of the body physiology of the patient with the trained use of the physician's conscious awareness and his sense of touch and palpation.

Rhythmic balanced interchange technique requires that the physician has a working philosophy and a physiological knowledge of the anatomicophysiological mechanisms of the body physiology of the patient. Rhythmic balanced interchange techniques in body physiology evaluate and create health (health: unlimited capacity to function in all areas of body physiology), and they diagnose and treat to correct trauma and disease (trauma and disease: limited capacity to function in specific areas of body physiology specific for each traumatic or disease condition).

Basically, the physician is trained in anatomy, physiology, pathology, and all other allied sciences to clinically evaluate health and *to do* something for the patient with medicine, surgery, or other modalities to diagnose and treat trauma and disease. Rhythmic balanced interchange techniques require that the physician goes another step deeper into the understanding of the body physiology of the patient by working *with* and *through* the anatomicophysiological mechanisms of the patient, utilizing the potency of the body physiology of the patient as the motive power to evaluate and create health and to diagnose and correct existing trauma and disease.

Life is movement in space and time relationships from the highest spiritual manifestations down to the simplest physical phenomena.

Body physiology is movement in space and time relationships from the highest spiritual manifestations down to the simplest physical phenomena. Body physiology involves energies at all levels of its existence in movement and time/space coordinates; it involves all the body fluids, all the soft tissues, all the osseous tissues; it involves interchange between all elements of body physiology from the highest spiritual manifestations down to the simplest of physical and environmental phenomena. It begins with the inception of the fertilized ovum through to the eventual sentient transition of the individual to another plane of action.

Each individual body physiology is endowed with potency, power, and energy fields to manifest life (movement :: space/time, highest spiritual manifestations to physical phenomena)—a potency that can be tapped, read, worked with, utilized by the physician in his diagnostic and treatment program to create health and to dissipate the effects of trauma and disease within the individual body physiology of the patient. Potency and body physiology are one unit of function in life's individual entity of being, and all levels of energy in the anatomicophysiological mechanisms of the patient are available for use.

Potency is more than a static value representing the potential of energy available to use. Potency is an energy in action from the simplest physical action phenomena to the highest spiritual manifestation. It is an automatic shifting entity of function in the balanced area of all rhythmic balanced interchange mechanisms.

Potency can be described in many ways. Potency is in the space between two notes in a musical scale that makes it possible for there to be notes of different quality. Potency will be found between different manifesting wavelengths of energy involved in electromagnetic force fields. Potency is between the ebb and flow of the tides of the ocean and the tides of universal energy in the solar system and beyond. In chemistry, potency is found at the sites of interchange between all chemical reactions. The potency at the "stillness" of the fulcrum is the sum total of all the energies manifested at both ends of the levers. The fulcrum can be shifted, yet it remains "still" in its leverage function; it is the site of the potency for rhythmic balanced interchange action taking place in the lever.

Body physiology demonstrates all the above-named examples (the action of speaking, electrical activity of the nervous systems, tide-like movements of the cerebrospinal fluid fluctuation, chemical interchange for hormones, enzymes, fluids, et cetera, leverages for musculoskeletal activities) and many more in its anatomicophysiological mechanisms. These are available for the physician's clinical use in the patient. The physician can train his sense of touch and palpation to work *with* life's movement :: space/time relationships in the anatomicophysiological mechanisms of the patient's body as they seek rhythmic balanced interchange in health or in traumatic or disease conditions. Simultaneously, the physician can develop his conscious awareness of potency at the area of rhythmic balanced interchange in anatomicophysiological mechanisms as he works *with* the body physiology of the patient in health and in traumatic and disease conditions.

Despite the apparent complexity of the descriptive analysis for rhythmic balanced interchange technique up to this point, KEEP IT SIMPLE. The body physiology of the patient has the resources to cooperate in all ways. It is up to the physician to learn to use them.

Definitions

Body physiology: total capacity of an individual to create health and to resist or adapt to trauma and/or disease.

Potency: motive power for life from the highest spiritual manifestations down to the simplest physical phenomena.

Rhythmic: the recurrence of an action or function at regular intervals; harmonious correlation.

Balanced: the principle of unity, of oneness; an automatic-shifting-suspension fulcrum within all anatomicophysiological mechanisms; the site of potency for all the energies involved in any movement :: space/time relationship; in it is the stability which lies in Cause.

Interchange: to give and take mutually.

Anatomicophysiological Mechanisms

Rhythmic balanced interchange techniques directly utilize the total energies and resources of the body physiology of the patient for both diagnosis and treatment through interpretation of life's movement in space/time relationships, including the interchange of the fluids of the body, all the cellular movement of the soft tissues, and all the articular mobility of the osseous elements. These techniques are more than fascial techniques, ligamentous articular techniques, or membranous articular techniques, yet these descriptive analyses of application are the working tools through which the physician can develop his sense of touch and palpation in order to utilize the total energies and resources of body physiology in a diagnosis and treatment program.

The simple lever and its fulcrum are used as an example of the movements in space/time of the lever arms across a fulcrum balance area containing the potency. In the functioning of body physiology, the planes of movement in space/time of the fascial and connective tissues become the lever arms in four dimensional relationships (length, width, depth, plus time) through which the physician can develop his sense of touch and palpation in order to work *with* all the fluids, soft tissues, and osseous elements of the total body physiology of the patient.

A.T. Still has said, "This life is surely too short to solve the uses of the fascia in animal forms. It penetrates even its own finest fibers to supply and assist its gliding elasticity. Just a thought of the completeness and universality in all parts, even though you turn the visions of your mind to follow the infinitely fine nerves. There you see the fascia, and in your wonder and surprise, you exclaim, 'Omnipresent in man and all living beings of the land and sea.'"[2]

Thus the physician has a living reference for his sense of touch and palpation for the total body physiology of the patient by reading, guiding, controlling, directing, and cooperating *with* the fascial planes of movement in space/time relationship for evaluation of health and diagnosis and treatment of trauma and disease *within* the patient. The potency provides the energies, and the four-dimensional lever arms of the fascias and ligaments provide the living movements of anatomicophysiological mechanisms *within* the patient for utilization by the physician.

———

2. A.T. Still, *Philosophy of Osteopathy*, p. 165.

Physician's Prerequisites

Detailed knowledge and experience in working *with* ana-tomicophysiological functioning in body physiology with a trained sense of touch, palpation, and ability to read the changes in function in health, trauma, and disease in a treatment program.

Knowledge and experience in working *with* potency in body physiology through awareness (consciousness) of potency at the area of balance in rhythmic balanced interchange and being able to be aware of a shift at the site of potency in health, trauma, and disease in a treatment program.

General Principles

The primary goal of the resources of body physiology is to create health for the individual. The tendency of body physiology is always towards health. When trauma or disease is added to body physiology, it resists or adapts to the limitations imposed upon it and continues to seek health in anatomicophysiological functioning. Rhythmic balanced interchange techniques are a direct approach to *work with* and *assist* body physiology to create health and to dissipate trauma and disease in its anatomicophysiological functioning. It is the intelligent use of rhythmic balanced interchange techniques plus medical and/or surgical intervention, if necessary, that will give the most efficient care to the body physiology of the patient in its time of need. The capacity of body physiology to heal itself cannot be overestimated.

Rhythmic Balanced Interchange Technique

This technique is a method whereby the body physiology of the patient can be made to evaluate itself as to its state of health and to treat itself for any trauma or disease condition that may be present utilizing its own resources together with those contributed by the physician. The application of this technique in action within the body of the patient can be monitored by the physician through the physician's sense of palpation and his conscious awareness of the tissue processes in their cycle of treatment. The available corrections obtained at one treatment session will carry through to the next scheduled treatment.

1. The physician chooses the target site for the treatment based upon the patient's history of his complaint and other tests the physician may run to determine that which needs attention first.

2. The physician positions his hand or hands upon the body over or under the tissues of the target site and applies a moderate amount of controlled *compression* towards the tissues involved.

2a. The physician has established a fulcrum against the body physiology of the patient.

2b. The physician's fulcrum contact, like all fulcrums anywhere in nature or man-made, is the site of potency. The energy in this potency is immediately available and used by the body physiology of the patient.

2c. The body physiology of the patient begins developing rhythmic balanced interchange activity in the involved tissues. This is palpable to the physician's sense of touch.

2d. The physician's fulcrum hand contact does not remain rigidly, inertly fixed to the patient's body. It is an alert, living, experiencing, still contact with the body. The physician's hand or hands are flexible as a quiet moving contact adapting to the changes taking place in the rhythmic balanced interchange movements within the patient's body. The physician's hand and fingers mold themselves to the changes taking place within the patient.

3. The physician's sense of palpation through his projected sense of touch and conscious awareness follows, shares, experiences, becomes part of the processes taking place within the body of the patient at the target site until the induced rhythmic balanced interchange action has reached the balance site for this particular tissue involvement. The physician can recognize this balance site for two reasons. The physician has induced action into the patient's body through his fulcrum hand contact with its relative stillness

and potency. The relative stillness of the attained balance site within the balanced pattern within the patient is also a quiet area of stillness and potency. The potency of the physician's fulcrum hand contact is similar to the potency of the balance site within the patient. The physician is consciously aware of the sameness of this phase within the treatment program.

3a. Potency is *not* an esoteric manifestation of some unknown force or forces at work. Potency is a factor of function in the cycle of action and reaction wherever found in nature (consider the potency in the stillness of the eye in a hurricane). Potency is a living factor of function in the cycle of inducing rhythmic balanced interchange in the body physiology of the patient; following it to the balance site; observing, sharing, working with, and being part of the shift that takes place in the potency at the balance site which is accompanied by a release in the pattern of the rhythmic balanced interchange activity in the involved tissues. As a factor of function, potency can be intelligently used by the physician in his treatment program.

3b. The physician supports the tissues through his fulcrum hand contact or contacts at the balance site in order to bring about the shift at the site of potency at the balance site within the patient and a release in the pattern or rhythmic balanced interchange activity in the involved tissues.

4. The physician maintains his fulcrum hand contact or contacts until he is satisfied, through his conscious awareness and palpation, that a shift in the potency has taken place and the rhythmic balanced interchange activity of the tissues involved indicates that the elements in the target site are releasing towards more healthy functioning within the body physiology of the patient.

5. The physician then moves his fulcrum hand contact or contacts to the next target site within the body physiology of the patient. The next site is determined by the specific needs of the traumatic or disease condition under treatment.

5a. The physician again establishes a fulcrum-potency hand

contact or contacts through which the body physiology of the patient can continue the treatment program.

5b. The physician senses the shifting of the first target site response in addition to that being sought at the second site through his palpation awareness, and he blends the corrections desired at the second site with those created at the first site.

5c. He carries the second site activity through the same steps as for the first target site.

6. The physician continues the treatment program through as many target sites as seem expedient or necessary for the treatment program scheduled for this visit.

7. The time it takes for a treatment session varies with each patient. The purpose of the treatment is to arouse the body physiology of the patient to evaluate its own health patterns and to treat its own traumatic or disease conditions with the resources of its anatomicophysiological mechanisms. It may take a few to several minutes to carry the first target site through the treatment cycle, but once the body physiology response has been aroused, the subsequent chosen target sites respond more quickly to meet the continuing needs within the patient's body. The available correction attained at the first site, when the potency factors of the body physiological tissues make their changes, acts as a stimulus to continue to make corrective changes in all other target sites more rapidly.

7a. The time period for a given cycle through induction to the balance site and beyond will vary with the tone quality of the tissues being treated. Healthy tissues will have a good potency with which to work and will respond relatively quickly. Tissues in traumatic or disease states are locally fatigued, and the permissible correction available at the balance site may be even more quick in coming because the potency is low. The next scheduled treatment session will find increased potency, less local fatigue, and a greater response to the treatment cycle. The body physiology of the patient will give the maximum response available and the most efficient response it has to give through rhythmic balanced interchange technique.

7b. Moving from the first target site to other target sites will cause the body physiology to call upon more and more of its innate resources. The potency as a factor of function is also being treated, and it, too, will be enhanced by the work done through rhythmic balanced interchange techniques.

7c. The physician should stay within the time tolerance permitted by the body physiology of the patient and allow the corrections made for one treatment session to carry over to the next treatment session. The corrections thus obtained will be absorbed by fluids, cells, soft tissues, fascias, connective tissues, and membranes throughout the total anatomicophysiological mechanisms of the body.

8. The day arrives when the physician can feel and be aware of the fact that the body physiology of the patient is competently active in doing its own continuing work of treating its target sites, with very little assistance from the physician as he establishes a hand-fulcrum-compression contact and reads the treatment cycle in the tissues. This case is ready for dismissal for the pattern of problems that brought the patient to the physician.

Body Physiology Response in Rhythmic Balanced Interchange Techniques

Rhythmic balanced interchange technique is designed to meet the anatomicophysiological needs of the patient's body physiology in health, trauma, and disease. Each treatment session calls for an individualized rhythmic balanced interchange technique designed to train the conscious awareness and the sense of touch and palpation of the physician.

The physician projects his conscious awareness and sense of touch and palpation into the body physiology of the patient:

1. To evaluate the given state of health of the tissues for the individual at the time of treatment—to establish an awareness and a palpatory sense of "What is health for this individual?"—this is most important.

2. To evaluate the specific tone quality of the tissues at the target sites of trauma or disease as to whether they are actually involved, chronically involved, and the apparent time element of involvement.

3. To evaluate the potential for the capacity for the improvement in anatomicophysiological functioning in the target tissues for an eventual complete recovery in health or an incomplete adaption in relation to the rest of the patient's physiological functioning.

4. To evaluate the reactive time it takes to invoke or induce rhythmic balanced interchange in the multilayered fascial, ligamentous, and/or membranous sheaths and cause them to seek their own area of balance for the specific treatment in progress. Inducing the patient's tissues into their own internalized organized activity is most efficiently done through using rhythmic balanced interchange techniques.

5. To evaluate the balance site of the area of rhythmic balanced interchange in the target tissues—to support the tissue response at the balance site—to be aware of and to sense a shift, a pause-rest moment, a "stillness," a modification of the potency at the balance site in the pattern under treatment—this is the moment of correction.

6. To evaluate the corrective change taking place in the target tissues after the available corrective phase has taken place at the site of rhythmic *balanced* interchange.

7. Steps 4, 5, and 6 constitute one diagnostic-treatment session for one target area using rhythmic balanced interchange technique. The sequence can take place in as short a time as one minute for all three steps, or it may take several minutes, depending on the complexity of the problem involved in the target tissues. The anatomicophysiological needs within the target tissues will dictate the time it takes to run the sequence of (4) invoking or inducing action into the target tissues, carrying them through to the balance site, (5) pausing for available correction at the balance site during the "moment of stillness," and (6) observing the beginnings of unfolding into a more healthy anatomicophysiological functioning.

8. The information gained through the awareness and sense of touch and palpation working with the anatomicophysiological needs

of the first selected target tissue plus the basic knowledge of anatomy, physiology, pathology, and specifics of trauma and disease known to the physician will guide him to other target tissues to be treated during that particular treatment session. Anatomicophysiological needs may indicate several correlated areas that need attention, or it may only need one or two target sites for a treatment session.

9. During one treatment session, rhythmic balanced interchange technique is far more than a random hop-skip-and-jump securing of corrective changes in various target areas. It is an organized effort by the physician to take the available corrective phase at the first target site and blend, merge, fuse, and compound it with the corrective phases of the rest of the target sites into a smooth synchronous functioning pattern for the whole of the body physiology within the patient to meet the anatomicophysiological needs for that particular treatment. The combined corrections thus attained will continue their action and carry through to the next scheduled treatment session. At the next treatment session, evaluations, and diagnostic and treatment procedures will have to be redesigned to meet the anatomicophysiological needs for the traumatic or disease process under treatment. All target sites will respond differently than before, and some of them will have to be changed to meet the upgraded pattern of functioning within the body physiology.

10. The goal is outlined in step 1: to achieve "What is health for this individual?" Every treatment is a *corrective* step towards health for the individual regardless of the number of times it takes to reach that goal.

Body Physiological Applications

Soft tissue pathologies: (Muscles and soft tissue organs such as the liver, heart, kidneys, lungs, et cetera.) This requires the physician to have detailed knowledge of the role of the fascias in providing supportive connective tissue mobility for the specific soft tissues and organs involved.

The physician secures rhythmic balanced interchange in the fascial envelopes for the involved soft tissue or organ(s) to restore their mobility in healthy physiological functioning. In addition, the physician secures rhythmic balanced interchange in the associated venous and lymphatic drainage, the arterial supply, and the autonomic nervous system controls for the organs involved in order to restore healthy anatomicophysiological functioning.

Ligamentous articular strains: This requires detailed knowledge by the physician of the patterns of function of the ligamentous articular relationships of the cervical, thoracic, and lumbar spine, the rib cage, the pelvis, and appendicular areas.

The physician secures rhythmic balanced interchange for the specific ligamentous articular strains involved and also for the associated tissues for venous and lymphatic drainage, arterial supply, and spinal and autonomic nervous system controls in order to restore health in anatomicophysiological functioning.

Membranous articular strains: This requires detailed knowledge of the coordinated and integrated patterns of function of the fluctuation of the cerebrospinal fluid, the motility of the brain and spinal cord, the mobility of the reciprocal tension membrane (dura mater), the articular mobility of the 22 bones of the skull, and the involuntary mobility of the sacrum between the ilia.

The physician secures rhythmic balanced interchange for the specific membranous articular strains involved in order to restore health in anatomicophysiological functioning.

Trauma and disease conditions: This includes any and all traumatic problems regardless of their simplicity or complexity, and it includes any and all disease conditions regardless of their simplicity or complexity.

This requires the physician to have detailed knowledge of the anatomy, physiology, and pathology, and the changes in the patterns of anatomicophysiological functioning for each specific traumatic or disease condition as it progresses from its onset to the time it is brought to the physician and through to its resolution to health or to adaptation in the body physiology of the patient.

The physician secures rhythmic balanced interchange in the enveloping fascias, ligamentous articular strains and/or membranous articular strains for the specific target tissues of each traumatic or disease condition in order to restore health in anatomicophysiological functioning. In addition, the physician secures rhythmic balanced interchange in the associated venous and lymphatic drainage, the immunological centers, the arterial supply, and the central and autonomic nervous systems' controls in order to restore health in anatomicophysiological functioning.

General considerations: Medical science has produced a limited number of medicines, vaccines, et cetera, that are specific cures for a limited number of disease conditions of mankind. It is producing a rapidly expanding armamentarium of drugs for temporary relief or partial control of these ailments. Surgical techniques are rapidly expanding to handle pathology in all parts of the body and to modify and control other pathologies that would otherwise become irreversible. Rhythmic balanced interchange techniques offer an added service in the care of ailments of mankind on three counts:

1. The body physiology of the patient will permit the intelligent use of rhythmic balanced interchange techniques to improve the resources of anatomicophysiological functioning at any time in any type of case.

2. Where medical and/or surgical care is the primary choice of treatment, rhythmic balanced interchange techniques will be a beneficent complement in the care of that case.

3. In a high percentage of cases, rhythmic balanced interchange techniques are the primary choice of treatment, and medical and/or surgical care will be complementary.

Summary
The physician's role in the use of rhythmic balanced interchange technique is a dynamic pattern of cooperation with the body physiology of the patient. The physician uses his conscious awareness and hands to actively choose the target sites, and he actively establishes a

hand-fulcrum-compression-potency upon the patient's body through which the body physiology of the patient can have a baseline from which to start its rhythmic balanced interchange activity. This fulcrum is also a baseline from which the physician can read the changes taking place in the body physiology of the patient. The physician participates, senses, feels, follows, shares, and experiences the activities of the body physiology of the patient as it goes through the treatment cycle. The physician selects the secondary target sites to secure the most efficient response from the patient's body in the care of the problem being treated. The physician terminates the treatment session when he feels and is aware of the maximum response that the body physiology wants or can make for that particular visit. The physician schedules the next treatment session according to the patient's needs as expressed by the results of the treatment program.

The anatomicophysiology of the patient is a great teacher. The alert active mind (awareness, consciousness) and hands of the physician will make him an excellent student when he uses rhythmic balanced interchange techniques.

Rhythmic balanced interchange technique requires that the physician consents to be used by the body physiology of the patient to allow physiological function within to manifest its own unerring potency rather than the use of blind force from without.

⇒ ⇒ ⇒

The following are excerpts from letters by Dr. Becker to colleagues.

I wrote the enclosed article recently—it represents a verbalization of accumulated data over a lot of years. If the phrase "space and time :: movement" looks familiar, you will find it in *Main Currents in Modern Thought*, Sept./Oct. 1970, page 20.... [In that issue is an article] I read by an eastern philosopher who was discussing the mystery of time. He said that both space and time are two aspects of the most fundamental quality of life—movement.

❧

...The enclosed article is my latest "blurb" and is a continuation of the same theme discussed in "Diagnostic Touch." I do not plan to publish it. I wrote it to bring myself up to date in my approach to health, trauma, and disease, and to provide myself with a summary for my continued use of an approach in diagnosis and treatment. I have already been able to gain further knowledge along the lines suggested in the paper and should write myself a supplement... (1972)

❧

I have made another revision in the paper "A Concept for Health, Trauma, and Disease." The technique name is to be changed to "rhythmic balanced interchange" technique. Why? All cells in the body have a philosophy and a purpose. They are automatically in "reciprocal" interrelationship. The purpose of any diagnostic or treatment procedure is to secure "rhythmic balanced interchange" in their functioning. Therefore, change all "reciprocal balance" to the above. (1975)

❧ ❧ ❧

The following is from Walter Russell, A New Concept of the Universe *(1989 revised edition, p. 146; originally published 1953). This passage appears in the appendix of that book and is quoting from another book by Walter Russell,* The Message of the Divine Iliad.

"I have but one law for all my opposed pairs of creating things: and that law needs but one word to spell it out, so hear me when I say that the one word of My one law is
>   BALANCE

"And if man needs two words to aid him in his knowing of the workings of that law, let those two words be
>   BALANCED INTERCHANGE

"If man still needs more words to aid his knowing of My one law, give to him another one, and let those three words be
>   RHYTHMIC BALANCED INTERCHANGE."

4. What Do You Do?

This is an edited transcription of a question-and-answer period at a Sutherland Cranial Teaching Foundation basic course in Tulsa, Oklahoma in 1988. The quoted faculty members are Drs. Rollin Becker, John Harakal, Edna Lay, and Herbert Miller.

Question: I've had the experience of getting my hands on a head, starting to work, and then looking up and being shocked that 30 minutes have gone by. Is this a terrible thing to do?

E. Lay: You won't harm anyone, but it does bring up a good point. People doing this work can get so enamored with this marvelous, strange wave of rhythmic goings on that they just go along for the ride. They're just enjoying it. It will not do harm and you can do it forever, but it doesn't get you anywhere.

I'd like Dr. Becker to comment on the difference between "riding the wave" and "treatment." There's something going on when he is sitting there working at the table, even though it looks like he is just sitting there. I want Dr. Becker to convey the fact that there is some degree of effort going into what you do while you're treating.

R. Becker: Over a period of many years in treating patients, I have kept working towards the establishment of a one-on-one relationship between myself and the patient's own life matter. If you take away your personality completely, take away your name, take away everything you own in life except that which keeps you alive, then automatically you are simply a body physiology at work. If I can work on a one-on-one basis in trying to understand what their mechanism is trying to tell me, then I will be guided by the type of pattern and the type of function that is within that patient. Their mechanism literally is in charge of things. I do not look for a pattern within that mechanism. I listen to the mechanism functioning as it is functioning when I get my hands on it.

I'll describe a clinical case to make it easier. A man came into the office, and he'd been having brachial neuritis for over 18 months. He was a tough young man, but he felt miserable, with headaches and a dozen other complaints. By the way, one thing I allow myself to do is to realize that these patients are going to be living for a long time, so I don't have to solve all their problems the day they come into the office. But after two or three treatments, I was aware of the fact that this man was not improving any. He hadn't made any changes at all.

Normally, the body physiology is constantly making changes, and so at each visit I ask myself the question: Did they or did they not make any changes since the last treatment? I accept the fact that the potential for change is actively present in every single treatment. I accept whatever change has taken place, whether large or small, and I don't worry how long it's going to take for the patient to get better.

In this manner, after about the third treatment, I finally realized that I was sitting at the wrong end of the lever. Everything had seemed to be happening at the upper end of his body. But nothing was changing. So I went down and checked his sacrum again, and the thing was so completely locked that it was impossible for it to go independently into flexion and extension. When I finally got around to test for it, I got one hand under the sacrum and the other forearm across the ilia, and when I asked him to flex and extend his ankles, the whole pelvis dipped as one unit. This meant that his sacrum was totally locked up in that pelvis. The sacrum could not move independently between the ilia. The sacrum was the problem, but where were all the symptoms? Up at the other end. Everything up there was complaining because they had to function against the totally locked pelvis. On questioning him, I found that he once had done some very heavy, awkward lifting. This had locked his sacrum right down between his two ilia so it could not function freely.

To treat this, I applied a hold across the pelvis, across the involved tissues, and worked with it utilizing the tidal mechanism coming down through that area ten times a minute. I crowded in on the sacrum and the ilia in such a way as to tease them, to say to them, "Hey look, we're working on you." The next time he came back in, I observed there was some function beginning to come back into that 18-month-old problem. Soon after, during another treatment, all of a sudden the pelvis shook, the sacrum went back to work, and he lost all his symptomatology.

The point I'm trying to make is this: We are guided by the living physiology of the patient to go looking for the place where there is something that can be done to allow his body to train itself to let go of its problems, and often it is not where the symptoms are. By constantly reading this living mechanism, we can know how they responded to what was done in the last treatment and consider what can possibly be done on this particular day.

There is a constant shifting availability of information. What does that body have that it wants to tell me, and how can I tease it to make it speak louder? How can I feel that something is going to happen, and all of a sudden I'm aware that it did happen, so I'd better let go and let it go home and get well? This approach to treatment is an organized method of allowing a human mechanism to make a change in a living body by a living physician.

I accept the fact that I can learn how to use this patient's body physiology to do its own work. The question is: What's the simplest mechanism I can use that literally has some control over everything in the body? There are many different kinds of mechanisms working. Think of everything our bodies do. Yet whatever it is doing, everything in the body is simply going rhythmically into flexion/external rotation and extension/internal rotation. Absolutely everything. I have developed palpatory skills with which to read the flexion and extension mechanism of any tissue of the body. I don't have to call it a muscle, I don't have to call it an elbow. I can just call it a part of the body that is obeying the rules.

I can work with anything in the body I choose because every tissue is following the rule of flexion and extension. It doesn't have to have a name. The other thing is that everything in the body has a fluid drive, or otherwise it wouldn't be working in the first place. So my palpatory skill can read the fluid drive that accompanies the flexion and extension.

Here's another clinical example. A woman comes into the office with a psoas muscle strain pattern you wouldn't believe. She was in a tent camping, and, in the middle of the night, a wolf had howled and her husband had popped up to see what it was and had put his elbow right in her psoas muscle.

In examining her, I first assess her opposite shoulder, not because there is anything wrong up there but because I want to know what her normal flexion/external rotation pattern is like and how her fluid drive functions. How vital is the fluctuation of the cerebrospinal fluid? Is there a pattern that is going through this area? How does it feel in health? I sense and read as carefully as I can: What is the health mechanism for this relatively healthy area?

Now I've got a goal. I know this is what I should expect to find if I ever get a correction in the lesioned area. It doesn't take long to make this assessment, two to three minutes, whatever it takes to literally feel and listen to the tissues there. Then I go to the area where the strain pattern is. I crowd in on the area, putting in some compression in the injured area, and I do not feel any of the things I felt up in the uninjured area. Nothing is happening in that area of strain. It can't. It's in strain, it's asleep, and it's been that way for six months. So I key into this area and get my hand around these tissues. Then I begin to crowd in on the area, asking and following it, and working with the fascia and the flexion-extension mechanism that governs that area. I'm going to tease around with whatever I can find to see if maybe there is something happening. After a few minutes, all of a sudden, I'm aware that maybe something happened, maybe not, but I'm going to let go anyway. Before she leaves the office, I'll check out the relatively normal area again and see that it's still working like it should.

I allow a week to pass before the patient comes back in. When she does, I go back up to the shoulder area and check that it's still working well. I then go down to the trouble area, and there's still not much going on, so I'll key in on it again. I work with it until I hear this little, tiny thing that's just barely audible, and it says, "Maybe I'm awake, and maybe I'm not." But I don't treat it anymore that day. Believe me I don't. You should never insult, through overwork, a tired patient, a tired tissue. You can work with it over time, and it will become less tired.

After the third or fourth visit, I'm aware of the fact that there is now something happening down there. The day comes when this working mechanism literally creates a change deep within the fascia. The fluid tide finally manages to work its way through that injured tissue.

The next time she comes back, her mechanism says, "I'm doing pretty good over here. I'm working out of this, so please let me skip any treatment for the next two weeks, and let me absorb all this." So I'm through for that day. The patient comes back, and I feel the same "life" down in the psoas that I feel up in her shoulder. Using my palpatory skills, I am guided by that patient with her fluid drive and flexion-extension mechanism as the sole tools.

It took me a long time to realize that you can keep boiling this mechanism down to its utter simplicity. There isn't a single medical textbook that says the total body physiology is a flexion-extension mechanism with a fluid drive, but every patient's body that walks into your office is one. You don't have to go shopping for it. It's right there in front of you.

Question: Dr. Becker, you were just talking about crowding in on that psoas lesion, and yesterday you were talking about the idea of being back out like a "water bug." Could you address these two ideas? How do they relate to potency, and how can those two things exist at the same time? Specifically, could you talk about the concept of crowding in versus getting back out.

E. Lay (to Dr. Becker): That's what I wanted you to talk about—there are times when you do use some external force to affect the internal.

R. Becker: I don't know that I've got an answer. The water bug idea is just an image I use. I've talked about the fact that there are various levels on which we learn to palpate. There is the sense of touch in our hands and the proprioceptors in our forearm muscles. In addition, we can be aware that we're receiving this information through the sensorimotor system in our brains. Any of these approaches towards the powers within the human body are automatically available simply by studying the mechanism as it exists within that patient.

The patient brings in a problem, something he is stuck with, so we've got to do something to try and help him out. Let's go back to the basic idea we talked about earlier, that the body mechanism is a beautiful, organized system of flexion and extension of the tissues with a fluid drive. If we take away all personality from the patient, what we have is a living, individual body physiology walking into the office, without a name, without anything else to identify him. He simply brings in something that has a problem, and everything in that patient's body wants some kind of help. Otherwise he wouldn't have called for an appointment in the first place.

I'll answer your question in this way: If I take the total personality out of that patient and realize that I am simply working on whatever he has brought in with him, then I've dismissed his human body as a personalized mechanism while I am accepting his body as a total pattern of function. I see that it has a total flexion-extension, fluid-drive mechanism that already has everything going on as he walks into the office.

One way I visualize this is that it's like jumping onto a train while it's moving, getting a hold on that train, and following the engine and coaches around. I'm not dealing with any personality. Instead I'm picking on this mechanism and working with it. I may find there's a little thing happening in the first coach and another thing happening in the second coach and a third thing happening in the fourth coach, and the engineer is giving orders.

I can be a water bug riding in the various elements that this patient brings in, allowing me to be an outsider looking in, and I don't get wet. I can move around and work with that tissue, in and around it, until it makes a clinical response. I am an observer. I can be a water bug watching things happen and step back off the train before it has gone too far down the track. What we're talking about is the care of a living body that ultimately never wants to see me again, and that's the way I want it. So, I've got to have a point from which to observe this magnificent something happen. The water bug idea is just a simple approach for me to have some control over what's happening. I use the water bug to give me a little insight into following the mechanisms of a living body that does not need to have a name or pattern.

H. Miller: I want you to notice that the whole time Dr. Becker was talking he was talking about a mechanism and not naming things. If you get all wound up in the fact that you've got to name something for insurance purposes or for any other reason, you keep yourself on the edge and in a quarrel with the whole situation. That's because you look at it, and you stop and analyze it. You don't live with it in real time. Do your work and then, afterwards, you can analyze it and name it if need be.

R. Becker: That is 100% right. When I am working in my office on my patients, I am going to use this water bug or anything else I can. It is a separate part of my practice life when it comes to satisfying the insurance people and everyone else. I work on the patient, and then afterwards I will report that it was a cervical somatic dysfunction at the level of C5 and turn that over to the insurance company.

J. Harakal: Here is another analogy that Dr. Becker has given. He says that as we approach the patient in our intervention—or cooperation or whatever you want to call it—there is a boat of life that has been flowing down the stream long before you came along, and it's hoped that it will be going a long time after you leave. All you're doing is getting on that boat to help steer it away from some of the banks so it doesn't get itself banged up too badly. This is another way of saying, "Don't take yourself too seriously because your intervention could put a hole in the boat." What you're there for is simply to help steer the boat. Realize that the river of life has been flowing in that person since conception and will go on until death.

Question: I'm still not clear about what we are doing. We are following the mechanism, and now we're there, we're at the strain pattern—we see it, we feel it, then what?

R. Becker: Then what? We put it to work! You grab hold of the tissues in and around that area and put a little compression in on the thing. You tease the body mechanism, which automatically is going into flexion/external rotation and extension/internal rotation, and you follow those patterns within that area where it ran into the rock. I put my hands in the area and apply enough compression through my forearms, or otherwise, to initiate some type of change.

E. Lay: He finally said it. He does do something with his hands!

R. Becker: I'd like to answer the gentleman's earlier question about feeling drained at the end of the day. When I was practicing in Michigan in the 1940's, I became aware of the fact, after I got into this type of osteopathy, that I was a little bit like a yo-yo. One patient would come in with more stuff than they wanted, and they'd dump it on me. The next patient would come in because they were drained dry, and they automatically took everything I owned. So, throughout the day, I was either being sucked dry or beaten to death. The next time I saw Dr. Sutherland I said, "Dr. Will, I'd like to ask you a question. I'm getting tired of being a yo-yo. What shall I do about it?" He said, "Protect yourself," and walked off. You have the right to protect yourself. Each of you has to work out a system that works for you individually, but you do have the right to protect yourself.

5. KNOWING TO TREATING

This is an edited transcription of a talk Dr. Becker presented to his colleagues in the Dallas Osteopathic Study Group. He gave this talk in preparation for his presentation of this topic to a larger osteopathic group in Austin, Texas, in 1967.

OSTEOPATHY IS A VERY difficult science to learn. If you want to learn it, you're going to have to study the basic literature of osteopathy. There are many good books on osteopathy, but if you want to learn the fundamentals of osteopathy as designed and taught by Andrew Taylor Still, you have to go back to his writings. Three of his published books are *Autobiography of A.T. Still, Philosophy of Osteopathy,* and *Osteopathy: Research and Practice.* To these books you have to add Harold Magoun's *Osteopathy in the Cranial Field,* because Dr. Still did not cover the detailed anatomy and physiology of the craniosacral mechanism in the same way that he covered the rest of the body. So Dr. Magoun's book is necessary if you want a complete analysis of the total mechanism of body physiology and anatomy.[1]

This does not mean you have to believe everything Dr. Still said. For example, in his *Philosophy of Osteopathy,* he goes into a lot of detail about the importance of ear wax. I never did know what he was talking about. In his *Research and Practice,* he gives all kinds of techniques for various disorders, describing how to make corrections, and I am not entirely in accord with all the methods he uses. I believe we have refined some of the methods that he used as far as

---

1. This talk was given before the works of Dr. Sutherland were published. See also *Contributions of Thought* and *Teachings in the Science of Osteopathy.*

analyzing, diagnosing, and treating "osteopathic lesions." It is not necessary to accept A.T. Still's approach in every circumstance as *the way* to do a thing.

Editor's note: The updated terminology that has replaced the term "osteopathic lesion" is "somatic dysfunction," which is defined as: The impaired or altered function of related components of the somatic system including skeletal, arthrodial, and myofascial structures; and related vascular, lymphatic, and neural elements.

For this talk, I chose the title "Knowing to Treating" for a definite reason. I could have also used several other titles—"Diagnosis to Treatment," "Principles to Application," "Anatomicophysiological Functioning to Anatomicophysiological Treatment"—because all these titles are about knowing. To merely think about a problem from the standpoint of anatomy and physiology isn't enough. You have to learn enough anatomy and physiology to literally know your way through the problem to the best of your ability. We never will know the entirety of anatomy and physiology, but we can know a lot more than we know now.

Among most physicians who practice osteopathy, there's a strong reliance on finding a so-called osteopathic lesion or group of lesions, getting in there and mobilizing them, and calling that a treatment. In a way, it is unfortunate that you do get results with that approach. You get results because the body tends to constantly readjust itself towards normality, and you've given it some help. This does not mean, however, that you've given service to that patient for the problem for which they came.

If instead of simply mobilizing the obvious lesions, you can gain experience in a set of principles, in your knowing, and in the art of palpation, you would know better what you can specifically do for this case. In other words, try to figure out in each case: What is the problem you're trying to reach? Why do they have this problem? After you have made up your mind on what the problem is by your examination, laboratory tests, radiologic findings, and your own sense of touch, then you give a treatment. This knowing-to-treatment is the ideal direction of flow in osteopathy.

However, when you start out, you have very little knowledge, and so you rely on the results from treatment in specific cases to teach you to know, and this is fine. In the early stages of learning osteopathy, you're going to rely more on "treatment-to-knowing" than you are on "knowing-to-treatment." As your skill and the results from your treatment improve, you'll gradually be thinking more about the knowing side, the principle side. You're balancing the knowing against the treatment, keeping your mind open to: "Maybe if I do this, this will happen." Then if the treatment doesn't produce results, you've learned by experience that it didn't work for that particular problem, and you'll readjust your sights and think of something else to do and maybe come up with some results. And when the next case comes in with a similar problem, you'll find you can rely more on your knowing in deciding what to do for them. In this way you develop your knowing-to-treatment, which is the ideal.

The osteopathic lesion has generally been the foundation on which osteopathic treatment is based. If we find an osteopathic lesion within a patient, most of us assume that this is probably the cause of this patient's problem. But not all of us in the osteopathic profession believe this is entirely true. Some of us think in different terms. When we run into an osteopathic lesion, we realize that the lesion is there for a reason. We try to figure out the influence such a lesion would have in this given area and consider the anatomy and physiology it represents. Perhaps we'll think back towards what could have produced this lesion. Why does this person have it in the first place? If we use the osteopathic lesion as a tool in our trade and not as a cause in our trade, then we are going to be using *knowing osteopathy*.

The osteopathic lesion is an effect only. It is not the cause of anything. The osteopathic lesion was produced by some thing or combination of things, examples of which we'll discuss later, and it represents an intermediate effect that we can learn to palpate with our perceptive touch. If we merely find an osteopathic lesion with our perceptive touch and proceed to mobilize it, we are falling far short of the importance of that lesion. It truly is only an effect. It is not the cause of anything. It's merely a phase of anatomicophysiological function.

The Factor of Time

All osteopathic lesions have four dimensions. Three of them we accept without thinking. We feel these lesions positionally in terms of the three dimensions of the body: height, width, and depth. But there's another factor in the osteopathic lesion, and that is time. How long has it been there? Osteopathic lesions, every one of them, whether the acute strain of 24 hours or the chronic lesion of 20 years, literally will tell you how long they have been present in that tissue. This is a matter of technical skill, perceptive analysis, and the sense of touch.

The sense of touch, as far as the osteopathic physician is concerned, is central. And it is possible to develop this sense, to learn to appreciate finer definitions in our sense perception. Through our effort, it is possible to gain the skills we need in our particular work. An artist, for example, can detect ten times as many color tones in a painting as an ordinary person. Musicians can hear sounds that we never hear as the orchestra plays a piece because they've trained their sense of hearing. We as physicians have to train our sense of touch, and we start doing this at a very late age. We don't get into osteopathic school until we're in our twenties, and it takes a long time to develop a sense of touch— a long time.

To learn about this time factor, you need to feel tissues, to read and palpate tissues, and to ask yourself, "How long has this lesion complex been here?" These are things that come only with experience, only with placing your hands on these tissues and listening to the story the patient tells you. Ask the patient, did he ever have this problem before? "Yes," he says, "about ten years ago." So you can feel what a ten-year-old problem feels like. Register what that ten-year-old problem feels like in terms of tissue feel.

Thinking Osteopathy

As a beginning student, you may run your hands down a spine

and say, "Oh great, there's a bump. It must be an osteopathic lesion." Then standing there, you wonder, "Now what am I supposed to do?" Well, you can question your patient, "How long has this been hurting you? Does this spot have any relationship to your symptoms?" Then you put your hands on their tissues, and you feel the relationship of their complaint to the feel of them in three dimensions plus time. What does this strain feel like? In this way, you gather a story of the effect that was produced by the environmental energy which has become an osteopathic lesion, which in turn is creating effects within itself in the anatomy and physiology of the patient.

Osteopathy is primarily a thinking profession, with a thinking diagnosis and a thinking treatment. There is no time at which you can quit thinking with every diagnosis and treatment. It's too easy to get into the slipshod practice of finding a strain, doing what you will, and hoping that it does some good. That isn't osteopathy. An old friend of mine gave the same osteopathic manipulative treatment to everybody that walked into the office. It didn't make any difference if you walked in with a sinus problem or a low back strain, he gave you the same routine treatment: right side, left side, on your back, crunch, crunch, crunch, popped your neck, and out you went. He had done it for 40 years and had made a good living. Had he ever practiced osteopathy? He had not. He's still a good friend of mine. It takes a peculiar type of mind to think anatomy and physiology, to correlate and coordinate the tissue pattern that we call the osteopathic lesion with the problem within the patient. And it takes skill—medical skill, knowing skill, and perceptive skill.

Most osteopaths think in terms of osseous relationships when they think osteopathy. They talk about correcting a fifth lumbar, a second rib, the third cervical, and so on, but this is the least important part of the osteopathic lesion in osteopathic diagnosis. I never had a skeleton walk into my office yet. Look at a picture of a cross section of the spine in the thoracic area and notice that the body of the vertebra is quite anterior, deep within the tissues. Notice the spinal canal with the nerve roots going out from it. The spinous process reaches towards the surface of the body, but observe the depth of tissues. Observe the muscles, ligaments, connective tissue, and blood supply to and from this total area. It is the total mass of this area that represents the osteopathic lesion, not the limited motion of facet arrangements at one or more vertebrae. It is the total mass of muscular-ligamentous-articular strain that represents the osteopathic lesion. When you lay your hand upon this patient, you are feeling all of that as a strain pattern, not merely the interrelationship of one spinous process against the other. This whole thing is the osteopathic lesion; it takes all of it to produce the osteopathic lesion.

The same principles apply to the physiology in the cranium as they do in the rest of the body. In the study of osteopathy in the cranial field, we learn about membranous-articular strains. We learn about the interrelationship between the dura mater and the cranial bowl. It takes the total pattern of membrane and bony articulation to create a membranous-articular strain.

The reciprocal tension membrane represents the connective tissue framework within the skull, and we can diagnose membranous-articular strains within the skull mechanism. Similarly, within the rest of the body mechanism, you have a complete connective tissue framework hanging from the base of the skull—from the point of the chin all the way around to the back part of the skull—going down through the cervical, thoracic, abdominal, and pelvic areas, and out from the thorax to the arms and down from the pelvis to the legs. This connective tissue framework is also defined into ligaments and other structures.

So you have a reciprocal tension membrane mechanism within the skull, and you have a reciprocal tension fascial mechanism throughout the rest of the body. Everything is in reciprocal tension balance. An occipitomastoid lesion can only be a lesion because there is a reciprocal tension in the membranes of the skull that permits that lesion to be created by force or injury. That lesion is maintained in reciprocal tension as a lesion mechanism. When you get into the mechanics of the body, the osteopathic spinal lesions are reciprocal tension lesions utilizing the connective tissue and ligaments along with the articulations to create a ligamentous fascial reciprocal tension mechanism. This is why you have to think through the depth of all of those tissues in analyzing an osteopathic lesion. Thinking in this way widens your scope of operations considerably.

I have pointed out that osteopaths tend to think in terms of osseous relationships; they are also oriented to think in terms of mobilization to secure a correction. However, mobilization is the least important part of an osteopathic treatment. We should think of function first and motion second. Why? The osteopathic lesion complex that you find within this patient represents the functional part of a strain pattern created by something, an environmental energy. Therefore it represents a reciprocal tension function pattern which is being demonstrated as a strain pattern, and unless you can analyze why it is functioning as a lesion, you do not know why you should treat it. Mobilizing a lesion just to get motion in it does not necessarily resolve the environmental energy it took to produce it. You may mobilize it and it may feel better, but very often, if you ask your patient to walk around the block and come in again, you're going to find the same lesion.

You have to develop thinking, feeling, knowing mental facilities and thinking, feeling, perceptive touch to feel function in this lesion area, to feel all the factors it took to produce this lesion. When you have all this analyzed, you are in a position to secure a corrective change by whatever technique you choose to try.

Range of Etiologies

Next, I want to discuss the osteopathic lesion in regard to its range of etiologies. There are physical, emotional, and mental etiologies, and we'll discuss each in some detail. Every osteopathic lesion has an etiology. It took some kind of environmental energy to cause it. Osteopathic lesions, as part of the symptom complex creating the patient's disorder, represent a phase available for analysis and diagnosis. If you're going to do a decent job of this, you're going to have to include the environmental factors that went into their production.

Just for the fun of it, think about each patient you see this way. When a patient comes in with a strain pattern, realize that this patient is a living, thinking machine; a computerized, highly technical motor system; a musculoskeletal and visceral system that has developed an osteopathic lesion as part of the syndrome or complaint that you're examining them for. Realize that their consciousness was involved at the time they developed these lesions. They were mentally present at the time it happened, and their nervous system was present. So think of their mind and their nervous system as you analyze the osteopathic strain patterns. You must include the environmental energy of this whole mind and body as well as the environmental energy of the external forces that came in to produce the lesion. Consider both the internal and external environmental factors.

Among the physical causes for osteopathic lesions, one of the first ones is birth. The mere act of being born can create two particular types of osteopathic strains. The first are the obvious strains of the craniosacral mechanism due to direct trauma. Fortunately, these severe strains are uncommon. The other types of strains are more important because they are so common and have far-reaching effects. These are more subtle, molding strains that are pre-osteopathic lesions affecting future growth and development. No one has a base of the skull that is exactly symmetrical in its anatomicophysiological function. There may be a slight curve into a sidebending-rotation or torsion, and the pelvis is going to tip correspondingly, so a mild scoliosis is going to develop even in the newborn baby within a few weeks' time, as the body mechanisms are beginning to form. Subsequent falls and tumbles can precipitate further pathology in these various areas. So one develops pre-osteopathic lesions just by being born. Think of how many pounds of energy from the mother's uterine contractions compress the baby as it is being born. These are energies that have been put into that baby's body.

From these birth patterns, you can get all kinds of scoliotic tension from one end of that spinal column to the other, which in turn modifies the relationship of the shoulder girdle, the pelvic girdle, and the upper and lower extremities. This creates a pattern such that in most people you will find they have an overall external rotation pattern on one side and internal rotation on the other side. This, in turn, creates somebody who in their job may have to use their arm in internal rotation on the side where they're supposed to have external rotation (in terms of fitting their normal physiological pattern), and this obviously can lead to pathology in that upper extremity. All these are factors you can take into consideration going back to birth.

Now let's go into something a little more obvious. Let's take trauma such as blows, falls, or strains from lifting, pulling, twisting, or pushing. In such a patient, if you confine your examination only to finding that osteopathic lesion, you have left out a very big factor in your knowledge. This patient is a thinking individual with a central nervous system, who had to pick up a pail of water on a slippery floor and reached over to do it. He thought his way through to reaching over and picking up this pail of water, and then his foot slipped. How many things were involved? The thinking process, the positional change when he bent over to get the pail, the weight of the water in the pail, the water on the floor, the direction of the slipped foot, and so on. All this is the environmental energy it took to produce this strain. The same applies to any kind of strain or trauma.

When a patient gives you their history, get the exact detail and visualize: How did this occur? What were they doing at the time? They say this problem first began ten years ago; what occurred then? What did they do at that time to lay them up for two weeks? Go back to the original problem and figure out their nervous system and the process they were involved in to create the living strain that is the osteopathic lesion you find in your examination that day. Most often, they're not going to tell you much about the strain; you're going to have to ask them questions. This doesn't mean you have to take a long detailed history before you start to find out what they are talking about. While your hands are on the tissues, get them to tell you the story. It only takes a few minutes, and it gives them something to talk about. You can feel what they're talking about as it relates itself through to your hands.

This approach gives you a lot more insight than just, "Here is a lesion." It tells you why their nervous system is involved in the way it is, how the pattern was set up within the nervous system. The nervous system must have recorded all this, otherwise these tissues would not be maintaining the fascial and ligamentous-articular reciprocal tension without some ongoing imprint behind it to maintain the strain. The body wants to correct itself.

Among other traumatic factors to consider are those of acceleration and deceleration, such as those that occur in all automobile accidents. Waterskiing and trampoline injuries can also impart this kind of force. In any kind of rapid acceleration and deceleration situation ask: How fast was the patient travelling at the time? How quickly did they come to a stop? In what posture did they go into the accident, and in what direction did they go?

Whiplash injuries are due to rapid acceleration and deceleration forces creating energy fields from the environment that are imposed upon body physiology. These energy fields are true energy fields. The patient has been hit by an automobile from some direction, and for a fraction of a second, due to the G forces, they weighed as much as 15,000 to 30,000 pounds projected in a given direction towards the point of contact. So it was so many pounds of energy in motion that created this strain pattern within this patient. You can feel this acceleration or deceleration in the acute case. You can feel the direction in which they're going, as an energy field.

Getting chilled is another physical cause for the production of osteopathic lesions. One time, a friend of mine was sitting in front of an open window at a meeting. He got chilled right across the lumbar area for two hours. He then developed a very acute psoas muscle strain pattern as a result; the lumbar enlargement of the cord had reacted to this chilling exposure.

Electric shock can also create strain patterns. I've experienced this in a number of cases, and I'll tell you about a recent one. This lady is 34 years old, and for the last six years she has found it extremely painful to lift her arms upwards. She has a lot of pain through the brachial plexus and down both arms. which began immediately after the birth of her first child six years ago. With this type of story, one could think of various possible causes, including a locked pelvic mechanism due to a difficult delivery or a strained shoulder girdle from pulling on the rope to help during the delivery. But her case seemed unusual.

I've now seen her three times. From my standpoint, the first visit was to find out that she was alive and had the problem. I put my hands on her and examined her to the best of my ability, and I found all kinds of osteopathic lesions in the upper thoracic and lower cervical areas, with a general tone quality of lesion pathology which didn't tell me a thing. In the process of trying to feel what was going on, I gave a treatment working to free up some of the pelvic restriction resulting from the birth process six years ago, as well as working on the area of her general complaints through the shoulder girdles and cervical area.

She came back a week later complaining bitterly that there had been no relief. On my second examination, my analysis showed that we'd apparently done a few things to eliminate some of the tissue pathology. With the changes that had taken place, I could now feel an area from T3 to T5 that felt inert; it felt only half alive. From T3 on up through the neck, it felt vital. From T5 inferiorly, the tissue felt alive; it had good nervous system vitality. But between T3 and T5, it felt as if it were sick.

I began to ask her questions. I asked if she'd ever had any bad falls, or if her head had been driven into the windshield of a car, something that would force this area into this severe pattern. No, nothing like that. Did she ever have an electric shock? No, never had an electric shock of any kind. But when I saw her today, she said, "You were right, Doctor, I had an electric shock seven years ago. A year before I had my first baby, I plugged an appliance into the wall and got a terrific shock that knocked me off the chair and left my arm numb and weak for ten days."

So here was the cause of her osteopathic pathology; for the last seven years, she had carried 110 volts right up through the cervical plexus and cervical enlargement of the cord. Her husband had re-minded her of it. This was the beginning of her pathology, although she had apparently gotten over most of the effects of it during that year. Then, after the birth of her child, with the sudden change of postural fulcrum which occurs in getting pregnant, filling up with a baby, and then subsequently emptying it in six or eight hours, the pattern had decompensated. It showed up after the first pregnancy, and it had been with her ever since. I believe it is likely that in time, when we can wash out the electric shock effect, there will be a chance to do her some good. We'll find out.

I have also experienced viscerosomatic pathology as an etiology for osteopathic lesions. I'm seeing a man right now, with an acute prostate problem, who has a major ligamentous-articular strain at the lumbosac-ral junction. Ovarian problems, sinus problems, whatever tissue or organ is involved, can reflexly set up segmental osteopathic lesion pa-thology at its somatic level of nerve supply. These are viscerosomatic lesions. I can never cover all the potential physical energy fields and etiologies that are available, but I have highlighted some.

Next, we can move into the emotional, psychosomatic, and men-tal reasons for osteopathic lesions, and here again we are dealing with energy fields. These mental and emotional factors within the patient can be of utmost importance. In the patient who is suffering from anger, his whole body is expressing anger—not just his mind but his total body. One's total body may be expressing fright or grief. This is a tremendous energy field. A girl who sees her father killed in an automobile accident has shock with grief, and it stops her menstrual periods for years. That's an energy field. Shock energy. Can that cre-ate osteopathic lesions? You bet it can. It can happen from any emo-tion you want to name. In my practice, I've seen dozens of widows who lost a husband they truly cared for, and grief is a very real prob-lem. A father came in once who had built a brand new swimming pool, and a three-year-old boy had stumbled into the pool and drowned. That man was in shock and grief, and he was locked from the top of his head to the bottom of his feet.

Under the category of mental activities I'll mention two, just to give you an idea, although there are dozens of them. High-pressure work is one of them. Day in and day out, a man is struggling to keep his job. It's exhausting to be at an office and be in competition with 40 other people doing the same thing. I've got a patient who is a trial lawyer, and I often joke with him, "The last time you relaxed, your mother carried you; why are you so tense?" He responds, "Because I'm a trial lawyer. I'm in competition with the opposing lawyer and with the court every hour of every day I'm at work." So mental work, the constant pressure of work, is a source of strain.

Some high-pressure businessmen take treatments from me on a periodic basis, not because there is anything specifically wrong but because I can return some of this energy field back to wherever it came from. Treatment can lower the tension pattern so that they can survive, do their work more efficiently, and feel better overall. Marital tension is another common source of strain. I see a lot of it. I treat one man once a month who is in a very stressful marriage, to reduce the overload of tension.

What we have been discussing are examples of primary factors in the production of osteopathic lesions. Osteopathic lesions are effects that are found in body physiology. When you find an osteopathic lesion, you must consider in your thinking these primary factors. Consider the energy field that was poured into the patient from without, and also consider the factors from within the patient, in their own conscious thinking and nervous system, that are leading their body to create this energy field. You've got to combine all of it.

Nervous System Responses

We all have studied the pathology of the osteopathic lesion. There is the acute lesion with its restriction of normal motion, inflammation, hypertonicity of the muscles, stressed ligaments, circulatory disturbances, edema, pH towards relative acidosis, and areas of facilitation from the nervous system. A chronic lesion becomes a compensatory mechanism with a well-organized reciprocal tension connective tissue framework to maintain that lesion, relative alkalosis, fibrosis, dehydration of connective tissues, and a continuation of the central nervous system facilitation.

Now here is something to think about. An acute lesion can be a segmental event at a local area of the spinal cord similar to a simple reflex arc, while a chronic osteopathic lesion involves thousands of messages flowing back from the tissues involved, going up through the central nervous system to the brain, and being imprinted as patterns of disturbance in that area of the reticular formation. Input also influences the related motor and association areas, which send messages flowing down again to those tissues. So you have a central nervous system arc as well as a local reflex arc. Then, if there has been involvement for any length of time, you've got hormonal and autonomic nerve system actions as well.

My point is that the environmental energy that it took to produce these strains is still in the tissues, along with the more commonly described change of arterial supply, lymphatic drainage, and muscle strains. The energy that produced this strain is still present, regardless of how long it's been there. I have felt energy strain patterns in patients 30 years after a whiplash injury. We have an energy field from the environment that is part of the strain pattern, and we have the living compensatory mechanism of anatomy and physiology which the body has adapted within itself to create the osteopathic lesion within its own anatomicophysiology—its own energy field. One isn't separate from the other; it's all the same thing. There's the anatomicophysiological energy of this patient's nervous, musculoskeletal, and hormonal systems, and the energy field it took to produce it. You have a combined total energy field to work with in dealing with these patients.

In diagnosing and treating these patients, you treat them as a whole in which the environmental energy and the osteopathic lesion are creating an anatomical pattern of dysfunction and you include the whole works. When they talk about this ten-year-old strain, you feel the composite energy of a ten-year-old strain being held there and maintaining itself because it's been there for ten years. Don't just feel the end results of the osteopathic lesion, but consider that the energy it took to produce that strain ten years ago is still there.

Clinically, in thousands of treatments, I have seen that by dissolving the environmental energy as well as by securing a correction in the anatomicophysiological component called the osteopathic lesion, the osteopathic lesion complex disappears for this given pattern of disability, and it does not return. Superimposed traumas may be totally released. The predisposed osteopathic lesions created from being born, when found in the adult, are going to be with them all their lives. The compensatory scoliotic patterns are part of normal living; they're very normal mechanisms. This is the person's pattern—they keep it all their life—and maintained in good order, it works, it's efficient, it's healthy.

I want to briefly discuss why I make these statements. Obviously I have learned these things, not from something I have read, but from the patient's physiology and anatomy as I have worked with them with my sense of touch. I have tried, and so far failed 100%, to convey this approach I am now calling "diagnostic touch." Nevertheless, it has been through this diagnostic touch that this information about environmental energy and all the rest of the things I've talked about have come through so that I can understand and make these statements I give you. The only reason I have any confidence in it is because it literally produces—I can explain why a patient has a problem, and I can do something about it.

Next, let's go back and look at the nervous system's response to the environmental energies superimposed upon this patient—whether physical, emotional, or mental—and see how this relates to our treatment. The simplest form of energy that can affect this patient is that forming a simple reflex arc through a segmental area of the spine in association with a particular strain pattern. Then there is a second part of this nervous system response involving more of the central nervous system. Here the message from the involved tissues—including the soft tissues and viscera—is carried by sensory nerves into the spinal cord and up to the brain. Many parts of the brain, including the reticular formation and thalamic areas, receive and process this information. And in response to this sensory input, we find a tremendous outflow of information passing down through the spinal cord out to all the tissues. So even with peripheral trauma, there is a problem in the central nervous system, and we have ways to help.

There are also effects that arise in the autonomic nervous system as well as stress factors from the pituitary gland and the hypothalamus. Hans Selye, in his book *The Stress of Life*, describes the various chemicals involved in the stages of alarm, response, and fatigue which occur in the patient as the stress syndrome. In one diagram, he has a dotted line leading from the site of injured tissue up to the pituitary. What the exact mechanism is for how these messages get there, he doesn't know, but he has shown central nervous system and hormonal system responses to environmental energy that have effects upon anatomy and physiology.

Interestingly, if you go back and read *A Basis for the Theory of Medicine*, A.D. Speransky brings out the fact that the central nervous system develops an imprint of pathology as it exists in the anatomy and physiology of the patient. One of his experiments demonstrates this point. He creates a chronic ulcer in the forepaw of a dog using caustic material and keeps it as an active ulcer for weeks on end and then finally allows it to heal. So for weeks on end, this sensory input from that forepaw goes back to the cervical enlargement of the cord and up to the brain and back to the paw again. Later on, after the dog is healed and apparently all right, Speransky provides a serious insult to the dog's opposite paw, and the original forepaw immediately breaks out with an ulcer again because that is the thing the nervous system remembered from the last time it was under stress. I think this occurs in our patients and is a big factor in the maintenance of the complexes we run into in some of our patients.

These thoughts should give you better insight into what happens when you use what I've referred to as the fulcrum point technique. In that approach, you lay your hands under a patient to examine an area of osteopathic strain and establish your fulcrum point; you get your hand against that tissue so you have a hand lever hold on the area you are examining. The patient's body mechanism initiates a response—the simple reflex arc, which is relatively quick—into the cord and out again. But it also initiates the responses of the central and autonomic nervous systems that go to the brain, participate in all the sensory interchange in the brain, and produce an outflow that finds its way back down through all these tissues. This occurs more slowly, taking a matter of seconds or minutes.

With your hand under this patient, you feel this gentle give and take, the swinging of these tissues. You are observing the responses of the central and autonomic nervous systems to this fulcrum point that you have established on this patient, and this tissue movement is coming from the body's anatomy and physiology. It is not the patient that is doing the moving. What initiates the total thing into motion is the patient's nervous system sending the orders down to all the components within this tissue mechanism, which is the environmental energy and osteopathic lesion. The fulcrum point of the operator has initiated this mechanism into acting.

When you establish a fulcrum point and then apply a little compression into it, you have an applied power, and it is the responses of the patient's segmental, central, and autonomic nervous systems that you are picking up as the tissues begin their pattern of action. When the mechanism starts into action, it tends to wind its way in towards the point of balance that's right for that anatomical-physiological-pathological picture. The mechanism comes to a still point, makes a change, and begins to unwind. Sounds simple. I wish it were.

Role of the Operator

Another important point is that the operator is not physically laying his hands on this patient in a nonvital, inactive way. You do not establish a fulcrum point and just sit there. If it were that simple, you could devise a way to prop a plastic arm under the patient, turn a crank, and go off and leave them. But the operator is part of this picture. He has invoked the simple spinal reflex and the complex central nervous system reflex, and then he observes the dynamic response—the anatomicophysiological changes taking place within the patient. He feels the adjusting fulcrum moving within the patient. He has to adjust the pressure at his fulcrum point to fit the case as it moves through its windup phase. His hand leverage contact controls, regulates, and follows the directions of motion within this process.

Only he as an observant operator can know when it has reached the point at which it has gone through its corrective cycle for that given day. The chronic fatigue patient is going to require less input to go through this cycle because they can't take too much. An acute low back strain due to a big heavy lift may require a tremendous amount of fulcrum pressure as well as hand leverage contact to maintain the degree of intensity of the energy it took to produce that strain.

We fail in our treatments because, like playing golf, we don't stay down with the ball. We look up, don't pay attention, and we don't get results. The operator is a dynamic living operator, and all the time that these changes are taking place within these tissues, he is diagnosing, he is asking questions of himself and of the patient. He doesn't sit there and go for a joyride, simply following the movement of these fluids and tissues and muscles and ligaments.

We often ask ourselves the question, "Why is an operator necessary?" He's necessary because he has to shift gears to adapt to the problems that are within the patient. And the reason he is getting a response in the first place within the patient is because he has invoked a segmental and central nervous system reflex arc.

I certainly could go into a lot more detail, but the substance of what I wanted to get across tonight is the fact that the osteopathic lesion represents a response to environmental energy, and both things together are a part of this patient's anatomy and physiology, and the patient requires diagnosis and treatment for both phases of it. This is true regardless of whether you use the fulcrum point technique or any other osteopathic technique. What matters is that you try to think through to analyzing the real importance of the osteopathic lesion, which in my book is a stepping stone for understanding the total pattern of physiology and pathology for this patient.

Recorded Conversations
with Donald Becker, M.D.

Periodically during the 1960's, Dr. Becker and his son, Donald Becker, M.D., exchanged tape recordings of their thoughts, questions, and news. The tapes from 1962–64 were recorded while Don was serving as a physician in the armed services in Germany. The later tapes, from 1966–67, were recorded after Don had entered private practice in California.

6. THE SILENT POINT

This is an edited transcription of a tape-recorded correspondence from Dr. Becker to his son, Donald Becker, M.D., in May 1962.

REB: The silent point is a tough thing to talk about. How do you discuss potency? How do you discuss anything that has to do with the fulcrum—with that still point? It is demonstrated every day in our lives, and yet how do you discuss it in a way that makes sense to those who are listening to you? Frankly, I don't know.

I called it "potency" in that paper for the reason that I had to call it something. In talking with a colleague the other day, I made the point that regardless of what terminology we choose to use, the fact is there is something that centers disabilities, traumas, and disease within human anatomicophysiology that carries the power, the authority, the potency for the pattern for that particular problem. Still it's tough to understand. You have to accept it more or less blindly, without too much knowledge of the actual mechanics involved.

Whatever words you use to describe it, it has proven itself clinically thousands of times. And if it works clinically, then there has to be some way to bring it into focus so that you and others can have use of it.

7. THE PRIMARY RESPIRATORY MECHANISM

This is an edited transcription of a tape-recorded correspondence between Dr. Becker and his son, Donald Becker, M.D., in May and August 1962.

REB: I'm going to talk about the normal respiratory movements, although they are not the movements people usually think of; instead they are the normal respiratory movements of a living homeostatic body. The ordinary respiratory motions begin sometime later after the "Breath of Life." When a baby is born, the first inspiration starts the breathing mechanism, the respiratory movements needed as we walk about on Earth. But even before the respiratory movements begin, all during the time the child is in utero, there is a rhythmic to-and-fro, ebb-and-flow, a rhythmic movement of every part of the body during the developing months. I am convinced that this begins right from the time of conception.

In order to understand the normal respiratory movements, we have to start at a period in life when there is no such thing as a lumbar, dorsal, or cervical curve the way we see it in the adult. We should visualize this mechanism as it is in the stage of the fetus in utero or at the time of birth. Dr. Sutherland described that during inhalation midline structures go into flexion and bilateral structures—including the paired bones of the cranium, ribs, ilia, and all the extremities—go into external rotation. During exhalation midline structures go into extension and bilateral structures go into internal rotation. This is the primary movement within every component of the respiratory mechanism. What is the primary respiratory mechanism? It is the involuntary capacity of the homeostatic mechanism to express itself during life, regardless of the postural mobilities of the individual.

The postural pattern in which there is a lumbar, thoracic, and cervical curve is a development that comes with time, with becoming upright. The basic pattern at the time of birth is that of a single curve that goes all the way from the sacrum clear through into the sphenobasilar junction. As that child breathes during inhalation, the whole spine goes into flexion—the base of the sacrum moves posteriorly and the coccygeal area goes anteriorly.

It is important to visualize the normal function within the total mechanism. It is important to recognize that, if it were possible to have a completely normal individual, one who did not acquire various patterns of molding strains, in utero or in the birth process, the pattern we have been describing would be the one in existence for us to observe. Visualizing the normal allows us to better understand the complications and the variations we run into in life.

DLB: We've talked about this phrase "primary respiratory mechanism" and its synonyms for quite some time now, and frankly I'm beginning to question one thing. Why is it present? You know what it is. You know how it moves. You know what structures are involved. You know its anatomy and physiology. But why is it there? We know a thumb is there to oppose, we know an eye is there to see, we know a foot is there to walk on, but why do we have a primary respiratory mechanism? What is its function?

Let me offer my own interpretation. It seems to me, from its very basic nature, that the primary respiratory mechanism basically represents the Breath of Life. That it *is* the Breath of Life. I can't think of any other way of expressing it. I think, perhaps, the most beautiful way it's been expressed is in Michelangelo's painting in the Sistine Chapel, where God is reaching out to touch Adam. If you haven't seen a picture recently, it would be worth another look. Mother brought home a slide from when I took her there. To me this painting shows me the meaning of the Breath of Life, the spark, so to speak. What do you think?

REB: Your last question is a good one. Why is the primary respiratory mechanism present? What is its function? And your answer is that basically the Breath of Life is the key to the situation. That is an excellent answer to a very complicated picture. The Breath of Life, the spark, the still point between the hand of God reaching out to the creation of Adam, that is the spark that initiates the functioning of the primary respiratory mechanism. The primary respiratory mechanism is this complicated anatomicophysiological unit that is responding to that Breath of Life. The functioning of the primary respiratory mechanism is absolutely dependent upon the Breath of Life, the still point, the potency. And whereas we define the primary respiratory mechanism in terms of its various units, a series of units within units, there is one basic pattern of motion, of flexion and extension during inhalation and exhalation, as a result of a spark called the Breath of Life, which is transmuted into function within this very complicated mechanism. Your answer is very good; it is sound, clean, and clear to the core.

When we examine the various units of the primary respiratory mechanism and find it doing its job anatomically and physiologically in a normal pattern, we are conscious of it as being in health. When we find some pattern of disability or loss of motion within it, then we attempt to restore the basic pattern that is right for that individual's primary respiratory mechanism. In doing this, we must take into consideration the fact that perhaps this individual normally lives with a sidebending-rotation or torsion pattern, and it is necessary to bring the external rotation pattern of one side into balance with the internal rotation pattern on the other side. This then restores the correct compensatory balance for that individual, allowing his primary respiratory mechanism to respond physiologically, as it should in response to the Breath of Life.

We find these compensatory, accommodative patterns routinely. We learn to recognize that this pattern exists within this individual as their normal pattern, a pattern which is right for them. When they are in a state of health, these various patterns exist in such a way that the primary respiratory mechanism is able to take the spark from the Breath of Life and function anatomically and physiologically in a total degree of health that is right for that individual. It is a deviation away from their normal pattern, which they have acquired or accumulated and which brings that patient to us for diagnosis and treatment. We seek out their normal pattern using the knowledge we have of what their correct pattern would be if it could exist within that individual. Then we work to bring it back towards normal, but always within the compensatory health pattern that is right for that individual.

It's a very important thing to get as complete a normal picture as is possible within human anatomicophysiology. There is an ideal normal, although we never see it. Nevertheless, it's still advisable to try and visualize the normal anatomicophysiological functioning mechanism, because even though we do not see the true normal, we do see within every individual a basic normal pattern that is right for that individual. You were born after a 30-hour labor and have certain cranial and sacral modifications you've had to manage with in your life. Each person has their own unique difficulties that they adapt around.

〜 〜 〜

REB: Actually, we cannot say whether the bone moves the membrane or the membrane moves the bone because the membrane is part of the bone—it is the inner lining of it. In addition, the whole dura mater, including the spinal portion, is filled with a fluctuant cerebrospinal fluid and a motile central nervous system. It is the total unit that is in motion, although in our palpation, we may focus on one part or another. We can gently turn the temporal bones and feel the tentorium cerebelli respond, or we can lift the membranes into their exhalation phase and feel the temporal bones rotate internally. But the answer to which moves which is that it is a question of the normal dynamics of this mechanism—the total unit is in motion in the normal mechanism.

When we get into the case where there are lesion problems, there can be a specific limitation of motion in which the membrane pattern becomes restricted and limits the motion of a given area. Alternatively, an articular lesion can exist in which there has been a blow on the head resulting in a limitation of motion between two corresponding bones, and then automatically the membrane attachment to the inside of that bone becomes limited, and by its connection to the membranous folds—the falx cerebri and tentorium cerebelli—the whole reciprocal tension membrane becomes limited in its normal motion.

In other words, if there is a blow upon a specific bone, we think of that as the bony mechanism having locked the movement of the membranes. On the other hand, the membranes can lock down the movement of the bones. There have been numerous cases where soldiers have been subjected to a lot of concussion by artillery barrage, standing under the guns of a battleship while shell after shell goes off overhead. This constant concussion is a shock wave that strikes their heads, reaches through, and bangs away at the cranial mechanism. It has not limited any bony motion in particular or set up any bony lesion, but it has acted in a concussive way on the dura mater, tending to lock the total movement of the membranes. I had such a case in the office recently. These men primarily demonstrate a limitation of the membranous portion of the cranial mechanism, and in turn they have restricted mobility in the totality of the articular mechanism of the skull bones.

The occipitomastoid lesion is a very traumatic type of lesion pattern in which there is a definite restriction of both the reciprocal tension membrane and the cranial articular mechanism—one of which I've endured or lived with most of the years of my life. This is a lesion in which a severe blow on the back of the head drives the occiput slightly forward in its relationship to the temporal bone. It usually occurs on one side only, although it can be bilateral.

⮑ ⮑ ⮑

REB: Don, you asked whether the internal and external rotation motion in the extremities is palpable? You also asked whether this is any help diagnostically once people have been injured? The answers are that this motion is palpable to a trained, sensitive touch, and I have learned to use it diagnostically in those traumas.

All bilateral structures externally rotate during inhalation and internally rotate during exhalation. However, due to the various stresses that we experience in the developmental years, there is a variation within all of us. The result may be a rotation of the pelvis or a rotation of some other parts of our mechanism. Because of these factors, for example, I can externally rotate my right leg easily, but it does not internally rotate very far. On the other hand, I can internally rotate my left leg easily, but I cannot externally rotate it far. So my basic pattern, due to my pelvic twist, gives me an external rotation in my right leg and an internal rotation in my left leg. As I inhale, the right leg goes farther into external rotation while the left leg, even with its internal rotation pattern, goes into external rotation; although the left leg doesn't go as far as the right because it can't. During exhalation, my right leg rotates internally even though it is limited in that direction by its external rotation pattern, and my left leg internally rotates freely. So even though postural changes and stresses have occurred, bilateral structures still rotate externally during inhalation and internally during exhalation.

Now let's look at this diagnostically. Most people are like me and have one side of their body in an external rotation pattern while the other side is in internal rotation. If in the normally externally rotated right leg I were to get a strain that would force the leg into an internal rotation pattern, I would have stress, soreness, or some other disability. My left leg is internally rotated as part of my normal, postural, general dynamic equilibrium, but I've added a strain to my right leg so that it is also in internal rotation.

I would diagnose this problem by going to the good leg, in this case my left leg. I would find it has a basic internal rotation pattern. Next, I would go to the side of the disability, and finding it also in internal rotation, I would assume that some type of strain has produced this internal rotation. I would then attempt to reduce or correct the internal rotation strain in the right leg, allowing its normal external rotation pattern to resume. This would restore the equilibrium that is correct for me. The equilibrium that is correct for me would still allow an external rotation of each limb during inhalation and internal rotation of each limb during exhalation. However, each limb would do so within its compensatory pattern, probably established during the process of my learning to walk about on Earth.

8. A DIAGNOSTIC CHALLENGE

This is an edited transcription of a tape-recorded correspondence from Dr. Becker to his son, Donald Becker, M.D., in 1962.

REB: Don, I saw a very interesting case today, which I think you might be interested in. A 36-year-old man was diagnosed as having a glioma of the pons. Currently, he has visual disturbances and a sense of weakness in the whole right side of his body. He first noticed symptoms six months ago with the visual disturbances and in about six weeks' time developed this weakness in the right side. He has lost the ability to coordinate his handwriting and has double vision and nystagmus. An interesting thing is that all reflexes are normal throughout the entire body. He's been worked up at three major institutions with X-rays, pneumoencephalograms, angiograms, spinal taps, and everything else, and their final diagnosis is that he must have a glioma of the pons. They were not able to visualize it, but they feel that must be what he has in order to explain this specific variety of symptoms.

He was sent to me by a doctor who has some faith in me as a diagnostician of the physiology of the cranium; he wanted my opinion. My examination revealed a very unusual problem at the base of the skull, so I asked the patient, "Were you ever in a car accident or did you ever have a concussion?" He said, "No." Then I asked, "Did you ever play football?" Yes, he had played football. "Were you ever knocked out in a football game?" He said, "Yes, I got an elbow in the face when I was making a charge which knocked my nose up towards one eye, and I was knocked out for a few minutes. While I was unconscious, they straightened my nose up."

I found a strain at the base of the skull involving the relationship of the occiput, the atlas, and the axis. The occiput and atlas had no motion between them at all, and the axis was bound down and tied in with the strain pattern in such a way that the odontoid process was in an obvious strain in its relationship with the atlas. Now what lies immediately above the odontoid process? The pons. And what lies on the anterior surface of the pons? The pyramidal tracks leading down to the musculature of the body. So it is perfectly possible that this very severe strain from 20 years ago, which locked the base of the skull, showed up six months ago with these symptoms. He could still have a glioma, but he also has a very severe strain involving the odontoid process of the axis, the atlas, and the condylar parts of the occiput which could be affecting the pyramidal tracts and the pons.

I do not know whether he's going to follow through with me or not, but physiologically speaking, it's an interesting problem. It was interesting to me to be able to find a traumatic pattern that physiologically explained the type of symptomatology this young man is suffering. I'd love to tangle with him for about the next two months and see if a change could take place in this 20-year-old problem, which in turn might have some influence on the symptomatology of his case, regardless of whether it is a glioma or not. They do not want to operate on the glioma because they cannot distinguish it accurately enough, and they feel there's more danger of killing him than there is of doing anything good.

Of course, I'm just giving you my initial thoughts. I've only seen him once, and I'm never impressed by my first examination of a case. It takes me at least three weeks to a month to diagnose as complicated a problem as this one.

9. A POINT OF REFERENCE

This is an edited transcription of a tape-recorded discussion between Dr. Becker and Ted L. Rankin, M.D., in August 1962. The tape was made with the intention of sending it to Dr. Becker's son, Donald Becker, M.D., who was in Europe in the armed services at the time. Ted Rankin and Don Becker were close friends and had been medical school classmates.

TLR: Well, Don, your dad and I have gotten together to develop this idea of his concept of a "point of stillness." He had me read his paper, "Diagnostic Touch: Its Principles and Application," in which he develops this concept and uses the analogy of the eye of a hurricane, and then he throws in other terms like "potency."[1] Well, when he first brought this paper out and we looked at it, you can imagine, there were a few points I couldn't quite understand even after we discussed them at length. Since then I've looked up some interesting articles and have come across some ideas that to me seem to make a little sense. Of course, I haven't tried these ideas out on your dad yet, so I may be drawing the wrong analogy.

REB: Let's start with whatever you found first, and go from there.

TLR: I came across this article called "The Clinical Value of Electromyography and Electrical Stimulation of Nerves," by Eaton and Lambert (*Medical Clinics of North America*, volume 44). I thought it

---

1.This paper was originally published in the *1963 Yearbook* of the Academy of Applied Osteopathy (subsequently renamed the American Academy of Osteopathy). It appears in an edited form in Dr. Becker's *Life in Motion*.

was pretty interesting in light of the previous discussions we've had concerning this point of stillness. Your dad defines a point of stillness as being a source of potential energy, and he goes on to say this initiates action or kinetic force. So with this thought in mind, I tried to find something that I could understand that might be analogous, something other than his term, "a point of stillness."

This article I found talks about the various types of abnormalities of contraction of the muscle. Using electromyography, they've defined a fasciculation as the spontaneous contraction of a motor unit or bundle of muscle fibers. While fasciculations are usually found in pathological conditions, they say they are found occasionally in persons who have no recognizable neurologic or muscular disease, in which case they are referred to as "benign fasciculations." The article reports that researchers observed that this form of twitching occurred steadily in healthy, young adults for many months, particularly in the calf muscles and in the small muscles of the hands and feet, generally after the young people had subjected themselves to an unusual amount of exercise. I thought it was interesting that the researchers say they are unable to clinically diagnose these fasciculations. I know that rarely can I ever discern a fasciculation grossly.

REB: What do you mean by a fasciculation? An occasional twitching of a muscle?

TLR: No, in this article a fasciculation is defined as a brief, repetitive discharge found in muscles of patients with tetany or other metabolic disorders, and these represent brief, tetanic contractions of a motor unit in which the action potential is repeated in a nearly identical form. Because a muscle unit is small, the contraction will not be manifest clinically unless you are doing an electromyograph at the time. But the tetanic contraction is something that the individual patient can feel or be aware of themselves. Eaton and Lambert go on to say that these contractions are limited in extent and do not ordinarily spread to involve the whole muscle.

I thought this was very interesting and might be analogous to your idea of a point of stillness, although this still leaves us with the inadequacy of the sense of feel or touch in developing this idea clinically. Don, I was telling your father about a patient I saw Tuesday night. He is a young, healthy male who was doing stockroom work, and he was pushing an object weighing approximately 80 pounds. He was leaning forward, the object was awkward, it tilted to the left, and he exerted a corrective force, which primarily utilized the paraspinal muscles. Immediately, he felt a sharp pain in the center of his back, which radiated down the back into his legs. He was able to straighten up and get relief, but afterwards, he had the onset of a dull, aching pain.

On my examination, the straight-leg-raising test created lumbar pain when either leg was raised. Palpating down the posterior processes of the vertebral bodies I found a central point of tenderness over the ligamentum flavus in the region of T12 and L1. Directly lateral to this area, in the right psoas muscle, I could feel a terrific spasm, so I placed my hand flat on that muscle. Your dad has tried to instill in me the idea of sensing what you can, trying to read the tissues, and I have to admit I couldn't read anything there in this way. But I did note a rather striking thing: In the center of this muscle mass that obviously was in spasm, there seemed to be an area about 15 centimeters in length and ovoid in shape, which was quiescent. I felt no spasm in that area. The apex of the oval area was directly opposite the point of tenderness on the ligamentum flavus. There I felt what I thought was an early, developing trigger point. There was a clear, focal area of increased tenderness. Below this trigger point was this quiescent area, the margins of which seemed to be composed of muscles in tetany.

I wondered if perhaps this situation is what your dad is talking about in his idea of a point of stillness and his analogy of the eye of the hurricane. This is a biophysical response that must be a potentiating area. Thinking of the Eaton and Lambert article, perhaps what we have here are a tremendous number of fasciculations with repetitive, ineffectual contractions that can be found persisting for several months, as those researchers documented. It is a central point and a potential area of further difficulty unless something is done about it. I have no idea whether your father will agree with me or not.

Regardless, I went ahead and treated the most tender areas. The trigger points improved, but I still didn't break up the area I thought represented a tremendous pattern of fasciculation with ineffectual contraction.

This idea of a point of stillness is a little hard for me to accept, and it may be wrong to try to apply the concept of fasciculations to the idea of stillness. But if we understand fasciculations as ineffectual contractions present for some period of time, then it seems it offers us a start on a physiological basis for this idea of a point of stillness. It could be a model that explains a center in which you can continue to have manifestations of disease.

REB: Let's go back to the patient you saw that had the acute low back injury. The quiescent area, the point at which you could not feel anything, was probably the point at which he created the strain. The points above and below, which you felt to be in spasm, were at the end of the lever. They were reflecting the irritation coming from that area in which you could not feel anything. If you had worked at that relatively quiescent area, not as you would treat trigger points but merely to make a change in the biochemical fluid dynamics of that particular area, regardless of what kind of change took place, you would have found a change automatically taking place both above and below that area.

I found some support for this idea in a short article published this year on nerve nutrients, which comes out of research done at the Rockefeller Institute in New York. It says that nerve fibers contract in a wavelike motion, carrying nutrients from nuclei in the brain and spinal cord. They suppose that nutrient substances not only nourish the nerve fibers but also perhaps the muscles at the nerve endings. They conclude that nerve fibers now appear to form a plastic, adaptable system capable of repairing some deficiencies or injuries.

In the case you are describing, the man has created a strain in a given area, which is sending stimuli back to the spinal cord and receiving, in turn, input from the brain—the thalamus and other areas—by way of the spinal cord. There has been a change of pattern within this injury which, at the specific point of injury, is relatively neutral, quiet, or still. But the involved muscle fibers extend above and below this quiet area. The psoas muscle has origins extending all the way from the twelfth thoracic vertebra down through the fifth lumbar, and then it passes through the pelvis and fastens into the lesser trochanter of the femur. So there would be irritable qualities above and below.

TLR: Now let's get back to this point of the quiescent area. You say— and this is the thing that gets me—that this is a strain area. Maybe you mean that this is an area of ineffectual contraction that can no longer contend with the amount of acute pathology it has been subjected to, such as the microtraumas and release of various substances that could lead to irritability.

REB: It's also in a kind of a state of shock at that point.

TLR: Well, it sure is, but my point is—and this is what always bothers me—this is sure not a point of stillness.

REB: Well, that does pose a problem, but suppose we were to chase this so-called point of stillness down to its real basic raw nature. Would you like to try to do that?

TLR: Well, I think that is where we have to go because what you're implying to me is that the point of stillness is a potential source of energy. Yet I think it's not a potential thing but an area of kinetic energy that's ineffectual—rendered ineffectual as a result of the damage.

REB: What is happening there no longer fits the pattern that should normally exist in a given area, but it fits the pattern for the area of the trauma. Let's say this point of stillness, just for the sake of argument, is the point of reference from which you can evaluate the rest of that pattern.

TLR: Well, first of all, was I right? Do you think this area I detected is, as you say, a point of stillness?

REB: Well, I didn't have my hands on it, so I wouldn't know. But if I were guessing, I would say, yes, that would be the point in which I would find I would do my work.

TLR: Then why didn't that area manifest some change that I could detect?

REB: It did. It was quiescent, signalling it needed help.

TLR: Why does the adjacent area, then, go into such terrific spasm, while this area seems to be blocked?

REB: Because the adjacent areas are at the ends of the levers. You said the irritability was at the twelfth rib, almost at the point of origin, and the area of stillness was down below that. It was expressing the irritability at the end of the lever, more so than at the quiescent point, where it was relatively quiet. If you could have felt the other end of that psoas muscle, where it attaches into the lesser trochanter—it's hard to find—you probably would have found equal soreness and irritability down there.

TLR: As I went down the psoas muscle itself, the pattern seemed to become more diffuse and indistinct, although there was still spasm there I could detect.

REB: Instead of calling it a point of stillness, let's say it's the point of reference from which you can analyze the picture as it exists above and below and around it. Of course you're dealing with a three-dimensional object there, but let's illustrate it here on this piece of paper in a two-dimensional plane first. I'm drawing a rectangle with two long sides and two short sides, and if I draw diagonal lines connecting opposite corners, we find the center of the rectangle, where those diagonal lines intersect, to be the relative neutral point for that given situation. Next I'll draw a rhomboid with the same equal-length sides, except now the two short sides are on a slant. Then I'll draw the diagonal crossed lines in the rhomboid. I have drawn the rhomboid underneath the rectangle, and if we drop a line down from the relative neutral point of the rectangle, we see that in the case of the rhomboid, the intersection point has been shifted.

The rectangle would be the normal pattern, which can get knocked in either direction and come back to neutral. But if a blow were struck at the upper end of this rectangle with enough force to create a strain

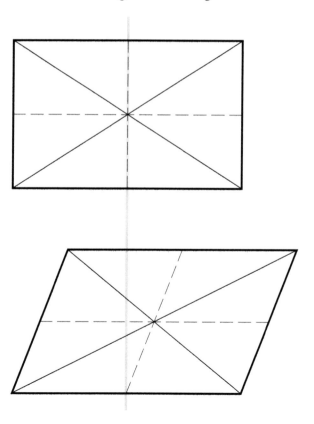

that could not resolve itself, there would be a shift of the pattern within the two-dimensional object. The trauma-induced rhomboid pattern that exists now wants to stay in this given direction. We find that this relative point of reference or still point has moved over. Does that make sense?

TLR: What about the compensatory mechanisms? I mean, I'm sure the body isn't going to accept things like this.

REB: In the body, things are three-dimensional. This is just a very simple, two-dimensional model.

TLR: Go ahead and try to develop it.

REB: Now on the other hand, if we were to draw a truly traumatic pattern in which there was a disruption of tissues, or multiple injuries, we could draw a figure that would have all unequal sides. In the rectangle and rhomboid, we were able to draw a line from the opposite corners and find one point of reference. But in this multisided figure, representing a more traumatic pattern, we would find variations, giving multiple points of reference. In the complex traumatic case that has gone beyond the point of simple strain and simple mechanics,

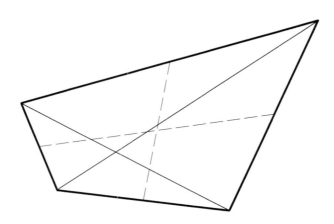

we're going to have multiple points of reference to represent this particular configuration.

TLR: Would it be proper to say that these points will also reflect the points at which lines of force or vectors of force are acting equally upon an area?

REB: Well, that would depend on the continuity of the tissues and what tissues were involved.

TLR: With these varying points of reference, I can see that if these tissues have reacted to some force or stress, the energy that has been invested in them, represented by distortion and so forth, is trapped energy in effect, isn't it?

REB: Yes, it's trapped energy.

TLR: And the mechanism for release, which may be over a long period of time, then could be manifested in the twitch which may be indiscernible to the clinician. And this would set up a pattern whereby...

REB: But the twitches that article is reporting are probably just the effects. They are the ends of the lever and represent the points out on the periphery. They do not represent these points in the center. They represent the points out here at the ends of the lever.

TLR: Let me ask you something. It may be that we're talking about the same thing but from different perspectives. Could it be that the point of stillness is what you clinically feel, whereas if we could record with an electromyograph, then we would perhaps discern that there were fasciculations or ineffectual contractions or twitching?

REB: Well, again I would say they're still dealing with the ends of the lever—they're still picking up the products of...

TLR: But you don't have a point of stillness until you have trauma or disease. Isn't this the premise?

REB [hesitates]: Umm...
Editor's note: This hesitation on Dr. Becker's part may be because in this conversation, he is using the word "stillness" in a way that is different from his typical usage. The inherent stillness in the body that he usually refers to is always present.

TLR: If you have normal, healthy tissue without a structural defect, you don't have a mechanism that's trapping energy or distorting it.

REB: That's right. If we were totally healthy–although none of us is– we would be responding uniformly to the interchange of energy that's going on within us all the time. In that case, there wouldn't be any trapping or binding or anything else. It's a constant in-flow and out-flow. It's only when we add trauma or disease that we get these localized areas that now have to conform to a definitive pattern that permits this disease or this trauma to exist as it does. The effect areas are on the periphery and the quiet areas are at the center of this pathology. The quiet area represents, more or less, a point of reference. If you could sit at that point, you could evaluate everything that's going on in that tissue. If you were a microscopic being sitting at that point, you could see the whole picture–the whole picture would be unfolded from that relative point.

TLR: That's an interesting concept to say the least.

REB: I think I can explain why what we are calling a point of stillness is clinically a point of reference. This point actually represents the total picture of the whole pattern–at this point the total picture is available. The other peripheral points are the effects. It's a point of stillness, but it represents tremendous kinetic energy.

Let us consider the physics involved, because actually, we're dealing with a problem in physics in all these things. Whether we're talking about human cellular structure or this table in front of us, it doesn't make a bit of difference—we're getting down to a discussion of energy levels.

Let's look at a given muscle cell, one single cell, which in turn is composed of millions of molecules. We have a cell and many molecules, but we still don't have a still point. Each molecule is composed of atoms, and the atoms are composed of a nucleus and electrons. If this molecule is one of the heavier elements, the nucleus would contain many neutrons and protons, and there would be several circling fields of electrons going around it.

All these elements are still expressing energy. Where is the so-called point of stillness within this thing? Actually it goes back to the physics of energy. The potential energy is located in the binding energy that is holding the neutrons and protons within the nucleus and supporting this electron field. It is not the neutrons or protons in themselves—they are expressing the energy.

We can take this energy concept and go back to our psoas muscle spasm in the biological sphere. We have said that in the injury there was enough force involved to change the normal pattern to a pattern of disability holding a force field off of its normal plumb or normal energy interchange. It is holding this energy at a given point—trapping it. The closer you get to the literal point at which this energy is trapped, the closer you are to the point of stillness. It's impossible to perceive it on a machine. We don't have the machine sensitive enough for it, including the electromyographs.

We pick up the distortions of energies as they are registering on the periphery, but we cannot register that point from which they are centering. That is a matter of knowledgeable awareness and an acuity of perception that you can develop. I can't feel a point of stillness, but I can sense by touch the area that represents the point at which this energy field is locked in this particular area. And I can also sense, spiralling from this point, the effects that we are getting at the periphery of this sick muscle.

If I wish to create a change within this pathological state, it is best not to fool around with the edges but to try instead to get as close as I can and create a change at this quiescent point. If I can dissipate or create a change at this energy level at that still point, then automatically everything else—the electrons, the atoms, the molecules, and the cell structure—has to change as a spiralling effect.

TLR: I won't argue with you; I don't know enough to. It does sound pretty logical that you have an energy transference whenever you have a collision. I believe this is accepted in physics. Now the big problem with this idea of a point of stillness is how will Don and I, without the clinical acumen you have, perceive this? How will this be manifested to us so that it will be of value in indicating that this is the center or, as you say, the point of stillness? In the case of the psoas muscle spasm, which I'm using as an example, I felt nothing in the center of that area, but I felt spasm completely around the margin. My question is this: You say I treated the manifestation rather than the point of stillness. How can I feel when I have reached this area in which there may be trapped energy to do something about? How do I perceive it? What are some of the basic things that I should look for clinically? Let's use the psoas muscle as an example because that is something we see a lot of in the low back syndrome.

REB: Okay, let's look at this point of strain in the psoas muscle. You felt the spasms up at the twelfth rib, and you probably could have found them down at the lesser trochanter. And somewhere in the mid-area, probably about the level of L2, was the so-called point of stillness.

TLR: Actually you're right. It extended from about L1 down to about L3.

REB: You can put your fingertips on the spinous processes and lay your hand so that the palm more or less covers this area of stillness in the psoas region. You have your fingers on the spinous processes as a point of reference, but actually you're going to sense through the palm of your hand. And then, if you apply a compression over this area of stillness, you discover that it takes energy on your part to match the amount of energy being expressed in this area of stillness.

TLR: What are the manifestations of this energy?

REB: As your sense of touch goes deeper into that area, it feels as if the area is resisting. It is quiet, yes, but it feels as if it has a protective wall around it, and it doesn't want to let you in.

TLR: This protective wall is not the same manifestation as the spasm at the margin?

REB: Oh, no. This is a wall of pure energy we're talking about. Put your elbow out here on the table. Now steadily push against my hand and I won't resist—I'll let you push my hand away. But if instead I push back with the same amount of energy that you are using, we will reach a point of balance and the relative force will be zero.

At the point of quiescence within this spasm, there is locked energy. As you compress in on it, you begin to sense that there's a resistance to this pressure that you're putting on. But you keep gently compressing in until you feel that you have balanced the amount of energy within that quiescent area. Through this action you have reached a state where you are voiding or tending to neutralize the energy that's within that point of stillness. In doing so, you have reached a point where *it* can make a change.

TLR: By my pushing on that, in effect aren't I adding to this strain?

REB: No. It's true you're compressing in on an area that's already in compression, but you're applying a regulated force. You need to have a sensitive enough touch to feel the amount of energy that is expressing itself as the energy field and compress in on it to the point where you can sense that it is now lying there being relatively neutral. It now has a relative force of zero, like when you and I were pushing our hands together. The odd part of this is that when you do move in on this relatively silent area, and you finally get to the point at which you have balanced out the energy field that's in that tissue, you'll begin to feel the ends of these levers modifying themselves. That's because you have reached a point where you can visualize both ends of the thing.

What I've just described comes from pure experience—I've learned to do that. When I'm sitting at the point at which I have balanced out the energy I felt within that sick muscle, I can sit there and read changes taking place above and below in that sick muscle. And finally, a change takes place underneath your hand within that point of quiescence. Sometimes it's just a little quiver.

TLR: Will this change be similar to those that I've experienced with you in the past? The change is almost imperceptible, but you feel a movement followed by a gradual warming type of feel.

REB: Right.

TLR: It always worries me at that point because I'm wondering if I'm wishing I was feeling it, and I'm wondering if I am fabricating it or tricking myself.

REB: No, you're not.

There are three kinds of motions you can feel. In the perfectly normal individual, what you feel is nothing. You feel the rhythmic interchange of energy, period. There's no feedback, there's nothing, it's just flowing in and flowing out.

Second, you can have a traumatic pattern. Using your psoas muscle example, when you first lay your hands on this traumatic pattern, anywhere in the periphery there's a nonspecific type of random movement. It's actually not random, but it's a purposeless movement. There can be muscle spasms and fasciculations—purposeless movement. You feel a contraction here, a motion there, a tug here, and a pull there, but it's a random thing. It can hurt here and then it hurts down there. It's a nonspecific type of motion due to the irritability present.

In contrast, the third motion is that if you get your hand over this area of relative stillness and start putting in a compression so as to balance the energy field within that area, you get a specific type of motility in which it literally seems to be winding in and winding out of this relative area of quietness. It feels as if there is an organized effort on the part of these peripheral structures—the motion is no longer random.

While you're compressing in on this relative still point, an apparent shift in the pattern takes place. You have been sitting there with a sense of the muscle pull or contraction, and then all of a sudden, this traumatic psoas muscle mechanism takes the pattern away from you. It literally starts winding itself. You lose the nonspecific type of feel, and you feel a specific pattern of motility. It's a specific type of motion now. It feels as if it is saying, "Hey, I've got a hold of this now, Doc. You just keep your hand there while I go to work."

Despite your contact and pressure, the patient will not complain. He will still have as much apparently going on, but it doesn't hurt him anymore. That is because now it seems to be coming in, coming in, coming in, winding in on itself, getting closer and closer to the center or the core of the specific pattern of this particular problem. After awhile, a little shift seems to take place clear at the bottom, at the core of the whole thing, and then it unwinds specifically again. That patient then clinically makes a change. If instead you were to lay your hands in that traumatic case at both ends of the psoas muscle where you felt irritability, you could sit there all day long and nothing would happen. It might feel good to massage it, but it won't change.

TLR: As a matter of fact, that happened in the case I described. I did just that, and he went out essentially the same way he came in.

REB: That's right. You won't accomplish anything clinically unless you get your hand in the right area, although you may not necessarily be exactly on the point of stillness because you can't always sense it. Sometimes in these heavy trauma cases, it's in shock, it's hard to find, but you do your best to try to find some area. You know for sure you are there if you ever get this specific type of motility—that's the only phrase I can think of for it—it seems as if this sick muscle takes this problem away from you, and it says, "I've got it." You get the sense it is saying, "I'm the boss now." It gives you that feeling as you're applying that little gentle compression. It takes over just like turning a switch, and you sit with that thing for a few minutes more as it works. Then that patient walks out saying, "Well, I don't know what you did, but something happened. It feels a little better."

TLR: Will these manifestations be present even in chronic cases?

REB: It's much more difficult in the chronic cases. With an old traumatic pattern, a lot of times you will work for many visits to arouse enough vitality in the tissue. It has been beaten down for so long that it cannot even develop either the nonspecific or specific type of motion. It has to be revitalized to a point where this type of motion can take place. In other words, this force field has gotten encapsulated; it is so well entrenched that it isn't inclined to make any change. You've got to revitalize it.

TLR: Do you think what has happened is that the force of the trauma or the illness has induced, in effect, a block so that you have poor electrical transmission?

REB: I think it goes back to the nerve nutrient idea we read about. They have found that the nerve fiber now appears to be a plastic, adaptable system, capable of repairing some deficiencies or injuries in muscle tissue. To me that implies it is also capable of maintaining that deficiency or injury. That nerve fiber is a pathway that travels clear up to the brain and back again. In these chronic cases, it can function like a broken record, playing the same thing over and over again until finally, through this work, you induce a change of pattern that registers up to the brain and out again. It's a question of arousing the total vitality of the nerve impulse and the whole mechanism.

TLR: That's interesting because in that article, Eaton and Lambert observed that by partially blocking a motor nerve leading to a muscle group, the muscle sometimes goes into these fasciculations or ineffectual types of movements. They also went on to say that in an effort to compensate for the number of motor end plates that were formerly available to fire, nature produces a branching out from the existing, functioning motor end plates. These branches go out to the adjacent muscle bundles that had been denervated, and what happens is that these muscles fire rapidly because of some physiological mechanism, and they fatigue rapidly.

REB: That goes along with what I was driving at in that paper of mine. I was talking in terms of energy fields in which the muscle, ligament, blood vessel, lymphatics, nerve supply, skin, and subcutaneous tissue are all acting as one unit. This unit is reflecting, manifesting, changing, and responding to the effects of trauma. I think you put it very well: It has these trapped areas of energy within it that want to maintain its pattern.

TLR: We've been developing this line of thought only in those conditions of trauma. How about where you have disease—for example, the case I spoke to you about of the acutely ill man with liver function abnormalities where we weren't able to identify a cause? I felt his liver and it was nondescript. I have never been able to really feel a movement of the liver on the falciform ligament as you describe. This altered function, was this either energy taken from or energy taken in? I mean, what would be the mechanism involved in disease processes in getting alterations, and how do you sense them? Do you have the points of stillness there?

REB: I believe that you do. At least in the cases I have worked on I thought I did, let's put it that way.

TLR: Did they respond?

REB: They responded. In the case of your patient, perhaps the trapped energy was induced by a virulent infection. An idea I have is that bacteria are smaller than cells, and they represent, from the standpoint of energy fields, a different frequency of energy. A cell will have a certain frequency of energy, but this little bacteria has a much higher, faster frequency, and a virus is smaller yet, so it has an even higher frequency of energy. So when a germ invades a cell, there's a modification of the energy field within that cell, which then becomes sick due to this outside force—the germ having entered from the outside. A modification of force has taken place within that lung in pneumonia or that liver in hepatitis. In the more acute case you can feel this, but when they've been sick for a long time, we again run into the problem that the thing has gotten slugged down to the point that it can't respond—it doesn't know how to respond. You have to work with it awhile to teach it to respond.

There's one point I want to get across before we run out of time on this tape. To me, this energy that's expressed at the so-called point of stillness is more or less trapped energy. If you can create a change at that point which represents that trapped energy, the whole pattern has to shift. There isn't any argument in my mind on that score.

But more important to us clinicians, if one could literally crawl into the area in a microscopic way and get to that point, one could see the whole picture of the disability. It is the point of reference—*Be still and know that I am* at the point.[2] At that point, this picture is laid out fully for me, whereas if I sit on the periphery, all I feel is this wind

---

2. "Be still and know that I am God..." (Psalms 46:10, King James Version). For Dr. Sutherland's discussion on his use of this phrase see W.G. Sutherland, *Contributions of Thought*, 2nd ed., p. 209.

blowing on me or that hurricane spitting at me. But if I can get right square into the center of that thing and have the correct kind of eyeglasses, I can see the whole pattern. It's a point of reference from which we can visualize the pattern of disability of this given trauma. I mean the words, "Be still and know that I am" literally—you do know. To me, that's important.

TLR: I'll apply it and see what I get out of it. It does seem important because so much of what we see—whether it's a minor or a major illness or mishap, like this back problem—are really problems which we in medicine otherwise don't have a good answer for.

REB: In treating this particular psoas muscle situation, I like to get the patient on his back and, sitting beside him, slide my hand under the flank on that given side so that his weight is resting right on my hand. With his weight there, I'm not working, his own weight is doing it. I also like to bring his knees up with the feet flat on the table so I can lean on his knees with my other forearm across them. In this way, if I put a little compression on his knees, up through the hips, I'm driving right back up into the psoas. And then I can sit there and move my hand, which is under the flank, up and down this area until I find the point of relative stillness.

I sit there and wait until his tissue either demonstrates a normal feeling of rhythmic motion—which you can always recognize by getting on the healthy side and seeing what it feels like—or a nonspecific type of random movement. If I find there's some altered movement, then I try to get to the point where this problem wants to take off by itself. Then I know I'm at least somewhere near the area that's going to accomplish something, both in diagnosis and in treatment. Then I sit there until I sense *a* change, not a total change, just *a* change. I look for this change not at the points of irritability above and below but at that point where this thing's crowding in on itself, and I let the peripheral ends take care of themselves.

TLR: After you have elicited a change, how do you feel about the use of moist heat to further dissipate what you've already started?

REB: I do sometimes suggest moist heat, or if they're complaining too much, I give them some aspirin or muscle relaxant, just to keep them amused.

TLR: But is there really some value in it?

REB: There is value in it because even though a change has taken place, this whole pattern has to change. Just because you create a change, the area isn't suddenly normal. There has to be a complete redistribution of this whole pattern. It's got to empty the lymphatics and venules; it's got to improve the nerve supply and wash out some of the old impulses.

TLR: So in spite of the fact that you have released the energy, you still have the need for recuperation.

REB: It takes time for healing. Also, in these cases of acute back pain, they've often hurt themselves before; it may be years ago, but this is their second or third go-around. So you're not only arguing with the current bunch of trapped energy, you're also dealing with trapped energy that has to work through beaten-down tissues. If this is the first time they have hurt it, they'll heal quickly, but if this is the second, third, or fourth time, it's going to take three or four weeks to heal.

TLR: We frequently fail to realize that damaged tissues put up barriers of fibrosis.

REB: Which I call "trapped energy fields."

TLR: I guess in effect they are. They've been walled off they've created compartments.

REB: Well, we're just about out of tape. Don, now it's up to you to find some questions and give us some answers to the problems that we've run into. I think we've managed to at least tangle with parts of this concept in a way that might make some sense. The difficult part of this process to me is that one has to develop a perceptual tool within oneself, not with an instrument. It's like the difference between a satellite going around the Earth with and without a man in it. There are so many things that the man, even with his limited sensibility, can pick up because he has the capacity to envisage past, present, and future. The unmanned satellite is only able to respond in a given, limited way. If we are going to do this work, we have to develop a set of tools with which to literally create an understanding of this thing, and that happens to be our sense of touch. It's limited in some ways, but it also gives more valuable information in a total picture than does any instrument, which is limited to the area into which it can reach. It requires a manned satellite to understand this work.... That is it. Good night.

10. ACUTE AND CHRONIC RESPONSE TO TRAUMA

This is an edited transcription of a series of tape-recorded correspondences between Dr. Becker and his son, Donald Becker, M.D., in 1966.

The original recording of Donald Becker's query is not available, so this synopsis is provided.

DLB: My question, which I had sent to Dad, was in regards to a 48-year-old gentleman who had been in a severe auto accident, with much thoracic, cervical, and lumbar trauma, without any definite fractures. The X-rays had been negative, but about four weeks after the accident, he developed a rather severe right bicipital tendinitis as well as nerve root symptoms on that same side. He also complained of pain during treatments. My questions to Dad had been, one, was I doing anything wrong in producing pain by treatment, and number two, why did he get nerve root symptoms without any evidence of arthritis or foraminal narrowing? I also made the comment: "I use the word 'whiplash,' but I dislike that word. If you don't mind, I'd prefer to call it an acute cervical strain. To me, descriptive as whiplash is, it's been bastardized so much that it has more emotional than factual overtones."

REB: Before I get into answering your questions on that whiplash injury case, there are a couple of other things which I will review for you because I have to discuss these matters from the anatomicophysiological knowledge of the tissues involved. I was reading in one of my science magazines an article on high-energy physics, and one of the quotations from Robert Oppenheimer said: "These papers, for all the variety, clearly reveal one common belief. All authors recognize that we do not understand the nature of matter, the laws that govern it, nor the language in which it should be described."

I feel that in the biological sciences, we are equally hampered. You have observed in my papers I've sent you the tremendous problem I have in trying to find language to describe anatomicophysiological functioning. It continues to be a problem as I try to discuss this functioning with you now. But my answers to you are going to be based mainly on what I have felt in tissues and on my interpretation of what I think that means in terms of tissue functioning.

I think the best way to illustrate this will be with your whiplash case, the 48-year-old man who developed a nerve root disturbance on the right side of his neck and arm. Your questions were: Why do these symptoms show up that late in the game? Why is he developing nerve root symptomatology without X-ray evidence of entrapment? My answer is going to have to go back to a physiological fact which I have become more conscious of as I've treated whiplash injury cases.

In spite of your objection to the term "whiplash" mechanism, I'm afraid that your "acute cervical syndrome" is just not big enough to cover the situation. The cervical area is certainly involved, but the whiplash injury goes so much further and deeper. There is a total shock to the entire body in these cases. The people are literally whipped with abrupt acceleration and abrupt deceleration. It is my observation that all three layers of the meninges—dura mater, arachnoid, and pia mater—are also equally whipped. They are a total mechanism which essentially locks itself down around the central nervous system—the brain and spinal cord. It is much like slapping the brakes on in a car, where they lock and don't release like they're supposed to. In examining these cases, I find a locking of the entire meningeal mechanism. This is in addition to the other findings I have described in the whiplash articles, such as the locking of the sacrum.

The dura is composed of two layers, an outer and inner layer. The outer layer forms the inner lining, the periosteum of the skull. It goes out through the sutures and blends with the periosteum on the outside of the skull. The periosteal layer of dura in the skull is continuous

with the periosteal covering for the inner side of the spinal canal, blending with the vertebral fascial structures all the way down the spine. The
inner layer of dura forms a sheath, which includes the folds of the falx
cerebri and tentorium cerebelli, with attachments inside the skull. It
fastens fairly firmly at the foramen magnum and the upper two cervical segments. The dural sheath then forms a tube around the spinal
cord all the way down to the sacrum, where it again fastens firmly into
the level of the second sacral segment. In addition, each of the spinal
nerve roots going out from the spine carries with it a dural, arachnoid,
and pial covering as the roots leave through the intervertebral foramina.[1]

With this information, I think we can find the explanation for why
your patient and others with whiplash trauma develop nerve root disturbances weeks after their initial injuries. I'll use another clinical condition to illustrate my point. In tic douloureux or trigeminal neural-
gia which develops after a difficult dental extraction, we find the
temporal bone on the side of the tic douloureux has limited motion.
The tentorium cerebelli forms a slip that forms a dural sheath around
the large trigeminal nerve where it rests in Meckel's cave. When there
has been a traumatic strain, we find that this dural sheath has become
locked in its functioning around the trigeminal ganglion. There is a
disturbance of the fluid interchange in and around that ganglion, and
there's a disturbance of nutrition because the dural membrane has
locked down. So eventually the patient begins to develop neuropathy
in the trigeminal ganglion and the symptoms of tic douloureux out in
the face.

I feel very strongly that because there is a locking of the total dural
mechanism in the whiplash case, there is a restriction of dural motion
in both the dural tube hanging around the spinal cord and the inner
periosteal dura, and in the dural sleeves of the nerve roots passing out

---

1. More recent anatomical studies have demonstrated that there are additional dural
attachments especially in the lumbar region. There can be short, strong anterior attachments to the posterior longitudinal ligament and weaker posterior attachments. The
dural nerve root sheaths are also attached to the posterior longitudinal ligament anteriorly and to the periosteum of the inferior pedicle laterally.

through the foramina. The free, normal motion of the dural mechanism—as well as of the arachnoid and pia mater—has been restricted in its function. So eventually, there are going to be nutritional disturbances affecting the nerves. This will not present as an immediate problem. The gradual nutritional disturbance begins to show itself as symptomatology several days or weeks after the accident. I think this perhaps could explain how symptoms can develop later on.

Obviously, the answer for eventual recovery is to take the shock out of the dural envelope, restoring its capacity to function as a moving, functioning mechanism, and gradually the nutritional disturbance will clear in these nerve roots. I've said there is a great deal of shock in these areas, but also when we use the term "shock," we're talking about pituitary and adrenal syndromes and a lot of other factors that enter into the picture. It's a matter of restoring the functioning capacity for a *total* mechanism, including the dural membranes, the locked sacrum, and the other involved mechanisms we specifically find in each case.

You had a question about an increase in your patient's pain with treatment. You said he complained of symptoms after the initial treatment and during the treatments that followed. You specifically asked: Do you go ahead and treat anyway despite the fact that the patient is localizing his pain, and is the technique wrong? I don't feel the technique is wrong any time you are restoring anatomicophysiological functioning. Treating in the area does affect the specific localized problems so as to allow the problem area to come back to life and to make the necessary physiological changes. Patients may have a lot of acute symptoms after the treatment, but then they were going to have acute symptoms in that area anyway.

So the fact that you woke them up to create a change is an indication to me that you did some good. If we're going to think in terms of anatomicophysiological functioning, we know very well that a sick tissue is going to complain. If you do something to a tissue that is not too sick, whether from disease or trauma, and it has a relatively minor problem in it, automatically it feels good. But a sick tissue that is told to wake up and make a change within itself is not going to wake up and feel better. It's going to wake up and be expressing symptomatology during the time that it is making normalizing changes. The more quickly you can secure a resolution of the pathologic functioning processes within any given area, the more quickly they're going to go through a normalizing process to secure healing in that area. So go ahead and treat them.

If patients complain they are hurting and want an explanation, I tell them that a sick tissue is supposed to complain while it secures a healing, and it is a temporary stage—and they will come through it in better shape. If need be, give them some analgesic and let them go on complaining and just work with them until you get the change you want.

The hardest part of this process of working with this sense of touch, this sense of analyzing tissue feel, this sense of working with anatomicophysiological units in the diagnostic or treatment program, is our interpretive sense—that is, knowing what the tissues are doing in terms of their functioning capacity. The only way to learn it is by doing what you are doing, using it in your practice in the cases for which it is indicated. Gaining that interpretive sense—the sense of analyzing function in terms of what the tissues are doing and are trying to accomplish, and what you have accomplished at a given time in treatment—is a very real problem for the physician. And it can only be solved by working with, feeling with, understanding with, and interpreting with your own innate ability, until finally the rules become pretty clear to you, and you gain insight as to their use. It's a matter of learning how the body responds to various types of problems and how to interpret them in terms of tissue functioning. It is also a matter of understanding the time involved for tissue change to occur for the pathology involved, so that one can assess treatment results.

⁂

DLB: I'd like to extend our discussion of nerve root symptomatology from that in the acute or subacute phase of a whiplash to a situation where the initial injury was untreated over a period of years. Currently, I am faced with such a problem in a good friend of ours.

The friend is 50 years old, and ten years ago, he was trapped under a car with a fair amount of weight on the side of his neck. He had been doing fine until about six months ago, when he noticed some neck stiffness. He couldn't turn his neck completely, but it didn't bother him too much. In the last two months, he has had numbness in the first three fingers on the same side that the automobile was pressing. The numbness is such that he can hardly grip or hold onto anything, which is a big problem because he is a maintenance man in a factory. He has some paresthesias but very little pain, indicating more posterior nerve root involvement than anterior. A cervical spine film shows intervertebral foraminal narrowing at C5-6. His pain increases with compression and decreases with traction.

It seems very likely that the symptomatology and X-ray findings at the present time are related to the original injury some years ago. There are now bony structural changes that account for this man's problem. Do you believe that these structural changes are a result of the nutritional changes caused by the involvement of the dura and pia in the acute phase? If so, can these impairments set up a compensatory response within the patient, such that there is an overgrowth of bone producing arthritis? Can these changes be prevented by correction of these lesions before they go into the chronic stage?

More pertinent at the moment is the question: Can this response be corrected or dissolved through osteopathic treatment? The answer is important because all the medical profession has to offer these people is neurosurgery, and, needless to say, this patient doesn't care to have his neck operated on. What techniques would you use to elicit a change to relieve the symptoms in these individuals? I have started him on cervical traction to relieve the nerve root pressure. I realize you don't agree with that approach, but at the present time, that's all I've got to offer him. Any recommendations you might have for the care of individuals like him would be appreciated.

REB: The patient you described is definitely an example of extending the concept of nerve root symptomatology through the acute phase into the chronic phase. In other words, he remained untreated for all the years since the initial process started, and this is the compensatory mechanism that has resulted. It's a mechanism that has tissue changes, arthritic changes, nerve root pathology, et cetera. Why the man had this pathology for ten years and yet only began to get symptomatology six months ago is a question I can't answer. It is possible he finally just got enough local problem up in that cervical area to be having some direct influence on the nerve root involved. Another possibility is that he has exaggerated this problem by doing something or other within the last year. Maybe he had another minor strain that kicked the whole mechanism into action and localized in the cervical area, where there was already trauma.

In answer to your question, I certainly do believe these structural changes are the result of nutritional changes down through the years. But to explain and understand it, we've got to go a lot deeper than just nerve root and dural pathology. We've got to go into the basic mechanics of tissue functioning, which is a total fluid balanced interchange between all fluids of the body. I'm going to go back to Dr. A.T. Still and quote him:

> What is the object of moving the bones, muscles, and ligaments, which are suspending the powers of the nerves and so on? A very common answer, is, to open up all the spaces through which nerves, veins, and arteries convey elements of life and motion. If that be your answer, then you have fallen far short of an answer that is based on a knowledge of the basic principles of life in beings, its method of preparing to repair some part, organ, limb, or whole system....we would renovate first by turning on the lymph, giving it time to do its work of atomizing all crudities.... Then we change the position of a bone, muscle or ligament to give freedom to the fluids with the purpose, first, to dissolve and carry away all detained matter and hindering substances, that nature can build anew the depleted surroundings.... We must know, if we would succeed as healers, that normal, does not simply mean to place bones in normal position, that muscles and ligaments may play in their allotted places and act with freedom at all times. But beyond all this lies a still

greater question to solve, which is how and when to apply the chemicals of life as nature designs they shall be.[2]

We can update this 1908 terminology of A.T. Still's using the last paragraph in the article you sent me on the mechanisms of death. The author says, "We can only speculate, but I'll look at all of this in terms of fundamental energy supply. A concept that appeals to me is that all of us, mice and men, are endowed at conception with a certain capacity for living, an inherited store of biochemical energy, if you will."

In my article, I have called this biochemical energy "bioenergy" and a dozen other things. More recently, I've been calling it "tide control." And when talking of "fluid balanced interchange," I am not only talking about the fluids that are circulatory in nature, I am also talking about an interchange between cells, between fluids, between anything within the body physiology, which includes the bone. Bone is fluid—bone cells are fluid when they are functioning. So when we talk about a fluid balanced interchange, we are literally talking about the living forces within this human body.

That little quotation from the article on the mechanisms of death talked of an energy in the body. In our work, we are learning literally to feel this energy, this bioenergy, at work. We are interpreting it as it does its work within tissues, we are learning to analyze it at work, and we are learning to use it to restore the normal templates of functioning, which have a tendency to be the dominant pattern within tissue pathology and tissue functioning. Even when there is tissue pathology, as in the case of your friend, there still is an underlying template of normal energy functioning. In the restoration process, we work with these tissues with our hands to restore that functioning by using the energy within these tissues to help them recreate that normal functioning. I only wish this did not sound so abstract because it produces clear results clinically.

---

2. A.T. Still, *Autobiography*, pp. 208–10.

You asked if the pathology could be corrected or dissolved through this method of treatment. Well, it cannot be totally corrected, but it can be restored to physiological functioning and become pain free, even though there may always remain tissue changes recognizable on X-ray and by palpation. But it is not a given that they must have the overlying symptomatology and functional disturbance. Another question you asked was: Can these changes be prevented by correction of these lesions before they go into the chronic stage? Certainly. If the lesion is corrected or the pathology is normalized, and normal tissue functioning can restore itself, they're not going to develop into the chronic stage.

Finally, you wondered what techniques you could use to elicit a change to release symptoms in this case. Regarding the traction you're using for your patient, I am not against it. It doesn't accomplish too much, but at least it's a step in the right direction. I would utilize a manipulative approach in treatment. You don't have to use the subtle approach of tide control that I use. You can use the type of functional technique you were taught by Harold Hoover, or you can use a technique which I'll talk to you about now.

Basically, you make a contact with all the tissues present and very gently feel for the pattern of motion, the direction in which they would like to go. In your patient with the sore neck, if you were to feel deep down into and through those cervical muscles, with your hands cradling his head and neck, you would be able to sense that the involved area tends to rotate more easily in one direction than the other. Sensing this, you very gently exaggerate the strain pattern, taking it in the direction that it likes to go. As you work with those tissues, keep that bioenergy idea always in mind. Feel for the tide that is deep within those tissues and try to sense that end point you have recognized before. Work with it until a change or sense of release seems to have taken place within the tissues. This only requires five to ten minutes for a given area.

To summarize, I would get in there and do a deep, searching study of the vertebral mechanics, the tissue mechanics, the muscle mechanics, and the fascial mechanics. Try to figure out what this strain pattern is doing in terms of flexion, extension, sidebending, and rotation. Evaluate those tissues as you put them through various moves, and try to find a point at which there seems to be a balance or a fulcrum point, where there seems to be a point of comfort. When you guide it over into that particular position, the patient, lying there on the table, often says, "That really feels good." This is essentially a fulcrum point deep within tissue physiology, and the patient is comfortable there. You then hold it there a few minutes while the tide and its mechanisms of bioenergy come into a focus. They create the change that *they* would like to make at that particular time.

In this type of case, I generally would treat twice a week for a couple of weeks to get the thing organized and then cut it down to once a week. You keep working at this interval until a definite tissue change takes place in those old chronic strains as well as some correction within them, and the patient begins to get better. Usually in a chronic case such as you are describing, within five to six weeks' time, there will be an appreciable change towards relief of symptoms. Traction is not enough in these cases because it's such a broad, empiric type of approach. You can do more for those cases with your ten fingers and two hands.

When you work in this way, every finger and every part of your hand in contact with those tissues is thinking through, and feeling and seeing changes deep within local areas. With your hands in contact with those tissues, you can specifically direct manipulative change or fluid change or tide change. You are specifically reaching in and towards a point of correction, which is certainly far more scientific than the mere application of a force from a machine you are hoping will do some good.

With the short amount of time left on this tape I want to make a general comment or two on manipulative work and techniques. I regularly have the question asked of me: What technique do you use for this problem or that problem? I believe it's always a matter of getting back to basic thinking on this. It's largely a question of knowing the anatomy and physiology of the part that's involved. If we're talking about a cervical area, understand the planes of motion that the cervical vertebrae would permit as far as the facet arrangement is concerned, and also understand the vertebrae's relationship to the anterior and lateral curvatures of the spinal column as a whole. Understand also the fascias and muscles involved, the 34 muscles of the neck and the fascial connections to the base of the skull and the upper chest. In other words, have the total mechanical understanding of how these tissues can operate within the area in which they are functioning.

You need to understand the anatomical, physiological, and biomechanical picture of the area you are examining, whatever part of the body it is. Then regarding the manipulative approach, you can get your hands on those tissues and carry them through the motions they can make, understanding with your hands which areas are tending to do what they are supposed to be doing while feeling for the areas that are not doing what they are supposed to be doing. In other words, you are analyzing the range of function within these areas, and then your so-called manipulative technique is to find the fulcrum point within the total pattern of change around which a given pattern seems to be operating. You carry it to that fulcrum point within the tissue, so that it can make a change of normalization or at least create a change within it which would permit the tissue to reevaluate its problem and to create a normalization. As Dr. Sutherland used to tell me, there is no specific technique—it's a question of understanding. If you understand your mechanism, your technique is simple. Your technique is your tool for utilizing a normalizing mechanism within tissue functioning.

11. Trauma Cases and the Power Source

This is an edited transcription of a tape-recorded correspondence between Dr. Becker and his son, Donald Becker, M.D., in 1967.

DLB: I have a particular problem in my practice situation. As the new general practitioner in town, I find it hard to tell new patients who come to me with chronic problems that they need to come see me once or twice a week for so many months. They are not used to doctors practicing like that, but I do believe that as I get some people who have faith in me as their primary physician, the practice along this line will improve.

One woman I did get to treat with a manipulative approach was a very interesting case. Initially I saw her in my capacity as an emergency room physician. She lives 20 miles north of here, and driving through town, another car ran into her right-hand door, snapping her head to the right. When I saw her, she was obviously in great pain, with a tremendous amount of spasm. Her head was tilted way to the right and could hardly turn in any direction. As the emergency room physician, I got the usual X-rays, which were normal, gave her some pain pills, and told her to check in with her doctor up north.

About two weeks later, she came to my office, saying that her neck was still hurting, and she asked if I would take care of it. So I proceeded to give her a treatment. I had my hands cradling her head, and then her head turned to the right and began to flex somewhat, just as though she was simulating the position that it went into at the time of impact. Interestingly, she was feeling comfortable the whole time. And I did as you suggested in your last tape to me: I allowed the head to go into that position to reach an end point, fulcrum point, still point, point of maximum comfort, whatever you name it, and I then felt it give. Well, she walked out of there with her head in almost complete freedom of motion.

A week later she came back and was much improved, although she still had some suboccipital headaches. I treated her again and the same thing happened. We shifted way over to the right, got into that cocked position, and it released and let go. Again, she felt much better immediately and left quite satisfied. I saw her again last week, a similar occurrence happened, but this time, her head did not go into the marked position it had before. She stated that she still had a few headaches and didn't feel just right, but when I thought of the number of whiplash cases I had seen who had not been able to do anything for three weeks, and here she was going around almost pain free, I was amazed. Incidentally, I also balanced her pelvis and did some work up between the shoulder blades. If you have any comments about treatment of these sidebending whiplash lesions, it would be most welcome.

I have another case on which I'm interested in hearing your comments. This is a man in his forties who, from a rather severe accident, has suffered a bad tear in his rhomboid musculature at the T5-7 level. I've treated him at least a dozen times now, concentrating on those right ribs, right rhomboid, and thoracic spine area while trying not to neglect the upper end as well.

He has a fibrotic knot in that thoracic area. It is sore to the touch, and when he uses his right shoulder girdle excessively, it hurts. It is now eight months since the injury. I'm trying to get it cleared up with what little I know, but we haven't gotten too far. He's a nice guy, and he's perfectly willing to let me work on him, so where do I go from here? Any comments would be most appreciated.

∽ ∽ ∽

Now I'd like to make a few comments, if I may, about what you are doing in both your teaching and your research work. I say "research" because that is in essence what you're doing. I've thought for some time about this and contemplated making these remarks on several occasions.

You, as I understand it, have been on the horns of a dilemma. Mainly you've been trying to write and teach this material in a language that people without your level of skill and experience may understand, trying to invent terminology and create phrases that allow an individual to actually get the idea of what you're talking about. It is an enormous task, trying to describe this type of material; it's like trying to describe the color blue. But I think this should not be your only task. The other side of the coin is that you should be forming a written or taped record of what you are doing, and the record should be in the terminology *you* want to use and that *you* understand.

This would have several benefits. Number one, you would benefit because you would finally be able to cut loose and say whatever you please. You would get some of this material down without filtering it, in the way you think it ought to be phrased. It would be as if you were just talking to yourself about it or to someone who is well-versed and can understand it completely. It would also benefit people in the future who could study this in the language which you yourself chose. You know they don't understand now, but it may well be understood 20 years from now with absolute clarity, or it may be transposed into the terminology of that era.

I do believe that someday, somebody is going to understand this work. They are going to have techniques available to understand the biochemistry, the power source, et cetera. Eventually there will be the techniques and instrumentation that have become fine enough to measure it. At that time, somebody is going to get some good from your descriptions. So I think it would be well worth your time, as well as enjoyable to you, to put it down the way you want it to be put down, as opposed to always directing what you say to those, like me, who basically know nothing about it and who have to transpose our medically oriented training and thinking into a completely new field. Though by all means, keep up that present work as well, because as far as I know, you're one of the very few who are making an honest effort to bring this stuff out, and it's going to pay off some day, Dad. I honestly believe it will.

REB: You talk about having difficulties as a newcomer because not many consider you their primary physician yet. Well, Don, in my opinion, you are the primary physician every time a case comes into you for help because otherwise they wouldn't be coming to you. Every case that comes to me for help has already been to many physicians, but now they are seeking my advice for this given problem. Therefore, for the time they are with me, they are my patient for me to try to understand and to deal with.

The next point is that people come to me for a particular problem, seeking symptomatic relief from that problem. They are really not coming to me for the total care it would take to follow the situation through until it is completely well. For example, a man came in who had torn and ruptured one of his thigh muscles in a bad fall three months ago, and he had strained his lower back in the same accident. He was having a lot of backache and of course a very sore leg. But the only thing he wanted relief from was to get rid of some of that backache. I gave him a few treatments, and his comment was that his back was feeling much better and that he would be in contact with me the next time he ran into trouble.

Now, this man still had plenty of trouble, both in his back and in his leg, and he has an awful lot of healing to do. The treatments I use would materially improve the quality and shorten the length of that healing period. But that isn't what he came for; he came to get rid of a backache. So I gave him as much treatment as was necessary to give him the relief he wanted, and he went on his merry way. In my opinion, he should have stayed with me, but in his opinion, this is all he came for. I strongly believe that 99 out of 100 of your patients who come to you for these chronic problems are seeking symptomatic relief. That's all they are seeking from me—a recompensation for their strain pattern to the point of comfort, and then they want to let it go until the next time.

However, I wish to make this comment: Since we are all merely patterns of compensation, it is not necessary to make a big deal in trying to do any more than the patient wants. It's fine to recompensate the case or the tissue to the point at which it is in comfort and then accept this as all the care that is required at any given moment. In spite of the fact that most of my patients are coming to me only for symptomatic relief, I'm at ease because I know that every treatment I give is corrective to the whole mechanism in addition to giving symptomatic relief. I just have to accept that these patients are not going to stay with me to the point where I am able to give total care to their problem.

Regarding the woman with the whiplash, in which you got such tremendous results, this is par for the course in the acute problem. I'm very happy you had a chance to treat an acute problem and feel the forces working as actively as they do. They are working equally as actively in all chronic cases, but on a much more subtle basis.

When you start applying this basic touch, you're going to find out that in all whiplash cases there are vectors of force towards the point of impact in addition to physiological changes within the tissues. When you went through the still point or end point in each treatment with that woman, these force factors were being resolved along with the physiological changes in the tissues. This is one of the big reasons for the speed of her recovery. These force fields were being resolved so rapidly, she did not have to carry them around with her, month in and month out as other cases have to. In other words, she was getting back into the physiological biosphere of her own being and was not having to carry around a unidirectional force vector field like a ball and chain dragging along after her through life.

I've observed this so many times. It's always an interesting observation to feel those force fields flowing out from the patient towards the point of impact and then, during the course of a treatment, begin to resolve themselves. In some cases, I have felt the forces flow right back into the normal biosphere of that patient, leaving the patient lying on the table with no further sense of outward thrust in any given direction due to an impact accident.

Now, for comment on the man in his forties with the rhomboid injury. When physiological processes have become pathological, such as this muscle damage which became fibrotic, the changes you hope to make towards normalization are going to depend on the percentage of reversible pathology available for healing within that situation. The reason we get results in any case, in the physiological care of our patients, is because of the potential for reversibility of the pathology in the tissue we are working on. Even though he has a fibrotic area, it is possible to promote some degree of reversibility with absorption of some of the fibrosis. This would make for a more normal musculature so that he does not have the pain and discomfort he has at this time. This will take time because fibrotic tissues do not have the rich interchange of healing forces as does an area that does not have fibrosis.

The goal of treatment in this man is to dissolve the fibrotic areas so that the basic template of normalization can come through and make for a more normal physiology. Specifically, I want you to do this: Put your hands under his back, placing one hand just below the area of the major fibrosis and the other hand just above the area. The hands are in fairly close proximity and compress in on that area of fibrosis. You are above and below the fibrotic area, and you have it as an entity of function between your two hands. Now, turn on the power, which I will explain in a minute, feel the change go through it, and work with it until you feel a change. Then you're through in that particular area for that particular treatment.

Since the man is having problems all the way from there on up to the suboccipital area, it's also intelligent to work on the entire trapezius muscle, which reaches from the suboccipital area out to the point of the shoulder and down to about T6 or 7. And of course you'll want to do some local work on those suboccipital muscles.

But you can do something for that fibrotic area by concentrating on it and turning on the power in that particular area during a treatment. You will be able to see a constructive change in a few weeks in terms of his gaining some degree of comfort. In a typical case like this, you may be able to discharge him in a month or two as the area gets comfortable to him. As this happens, he will learn to use his arm with some degree of feeling of health, and he will no longer have the binding sensation and the pain. But that is not the end of the process. Long after you may have discharged him, the healing will continue. A year from now, if you were to examine that area, you would find much less fibrosis because the healing process gradually normalizes the problem after you have given it the power to release its reversibility of pathology towards normalization. Tissues heal in their own time and place; we set them into motion to do so.

Well, these are my comments on your two cases and on being a primary physician.

Power Source

Next, I want to give you a brief lesson in basic touch. Since it involves primarily research work, accept it as such, go ahead and try it, and let me know what comes of it.

We are endowed with, surrounded by, and are part of a biosphere. In other words, my body is wandering through its time and place in this world of 1967, surrounded by a biosphere of activity which is keeping me alive, including a *power source*. Where is that power source? I know not, and it isn't important, but it is there. It is around you, and it is around each and every patient who comes into your office.

Now, just for the fun of it, let us imagine this power source as a cloud hanging over your office building. Make it a cloud above you. Next, consider that this power source or cloud can be compared to an electrical source with 110 volts flowing through it continuously. That electricity is always there, and it's always available, but it is being used or not used depending upon whether somebody plugs into it or not. Even if you do not plug into that electric socket, the energy flow is still there—it's working. If you do plug into it, you get specific use from that electricity. It's like having a tool, such as an electric drill, which has a switch you can turn off and on.

Now, you have a cloud over your head, which is an energy field in continuous operation, and you have a patient come in whom you are going to examine using physiological care and treatment. The patient lies on the table, you're comfortably seated, and you get your hands under the patient. Now, you're ready to go to work. Plug in the line to the cloud, just like you would plug in a line to a 110-volt socket. I mean, just like snapping your fingers—turn it on.

If this cloud were like a fluorescent light bulb and would turn on with a surge of power coming through it, who would be illuminated? Just the patient? No. You, the operator, and the patient become illuminated or have that power shone upon you. Both you and the patient are lit by that light immediately. Now, what happens? You, the operator, have your sense of touch turned on. Immediately, you have an intensified application of being able to feel what is going on in those tissues because your power source has been turned on.

Turn on the power source. Now, you can perceive better because you have turned on your capacity to feel. You, the operator, have been endowed with a surge of power. The patient's body has been endowed with a surge of power, too, and the tissue under your hand starts to go to work purposefully. The specific tissue that you have under your hand comes to life with purpose in its movement for the condition you are examining.

You can feel this purposeful movement turn on in tissues just exactly like you felt it turn on in the woman whose head cocked off to the right. In that case, it turned on strong enough for you to be able to follow it from its turning on to its treatment conclusion, which was a still point. In the more chronic case, such as your man in his forties, this purposefulness is not as obvious a thing, but it is equally dramatic at the subtle level at which it is operating.

That is enough on the subject. Before I give you mental indigestion, let's review what I've said. We have a power source. When I put my hands on a patient to make an examination and to treat, I reach up and turn on the power. My sense of touch is turned on as an operator. The specific, purposeful tissue response is turned on in the patient simultaneously because the same nondenominational, unbiased energy source turns on equally for both of us—the operator and the patient. Then, it is up to me to read that which takes place in the tissue under examination for this specific day and time.

If you want to have some fun with this thing and play with it, you can try this. Get your hand under some patient, establish a fulcrum point, and then reach up and turn on this power source, boom, just like that. Feel your sense of touch immediately be more perceptive than it was before you turned the power source on, and feel a purposeful reaction in a given problem. By the way, it will be easier if you try it on a problem that has a little vitality to it. Then, while you're still in contact with this process, turn the power source off, just like you would throw a switch to turn off a fluorescent light bulb. Immediately, see what you experience. You don't have to do this for very long; in 30 seconds or so you can evaluate it. I'm not recommending these stop-and-go signals on everybody who walks into the office. I'm just suggesting it for your own personal evaluation of this approach.

I presented this power source idea to the study group last week. How well it was received and what they're going to do with it, I could guess but I won't. Don, this actually is a way to improve your basic touch. That is the only reason I brought it up. Turn on the power, knowing that you are being turned on as well as the patient. Give it a little trial and let me know your response.

⤳ ⤳ ⤳

What follows are excerpts from two subsequent tape-recorded correspondences from Dr. Becker to his son.

I want you to do me a favor. I want you to go back to the last tape I sent you and erase all the information I gave you about "turning on the power." I was premature in giving that information to you without some other preliminary material. Also, I used a similar analogy with some of my local colleagues who are working with me, and I wasn't at all happy with their interpretation of what I was trying to say, their response to it, or their understanding of it. To me this means that what I was trying to tell you can be expressed more clearly.

⤳ ⤳

I'm glad you're using the power source. I also know that you got the tape in which I told you to forget the descriptive analysis I gave you at that particular time. What I said is perfectly legitimate in that when you get your hands on a case, you have to realize that your power to perceive by touch is awakened as much as the problem is within the patient. If you question the mutual cooperation between your hands and the patient, it creates a problem as to what you are able to perceive and understand. The source of that power is something we'll go into in more detail at a later date.

12. Levels of Palpation

This is an edited transcription of a tape-recorded correspondence from Dr. Becker to his son, Donald Becker, M.D., in about 1967.

REB: Don, I have two items I would like to share with you. The first item is from a foreword I wrote for some material that's going to be published. The second item is a brief discussion of the art of palpation. I came up with this thought in the middle of the night one night when I was trying to figure out how better to describe the art of palpation in determining function-structure and structure-function in anatomicophysiology. I'm hoping it will be helpful for other individuals who would like to train in a deeper insight into anatomicophysiology.

Here is the quotation from the foreword:

These works of William G. Sutherland, D.O., which you are privileged to read, illustrate the fundamental principles of osteopathy.... One of the principles of osteopathy that is so important is the fact that structure and function cannot be separated in the clinical evaluation of the patient.... It is an accepted dictum that structure determines function, and this requires very little thought or discussion to know that this dictum is true. It is equally true that function determines structure, and this idea calls for a far more searching analysis as to its full understanding in its clinical application.

During the formative time from conception to physical maturity, especially during the early months and years, the growing structural development of the body is going to have considerable influence on the functioning of the growing mind and body. For example, a physical birth strain pattern will influence the entire developing physical and mental pattern for the child throughout life. A scoliotic pelvis, spine, and chest cavity will cause a corresponding displacement of the organs within them and modify the functioning of those structures to meet the needs of the patient. Disease or traumatic conditions in the child's body, such as Legg-Calve-Perthes disease, will modify the functioning of the pelvis and resultant development of the postural mechanism during the rest of the growing period. There are hundreds of clinical applications in this thought.

However, after the body has matured in its physical development, with the modifications caused by disease or traumatic conditions, then function determining structure becomes the more dominant principle. Function-structure has worked hand in hand with structure-function throughout the formative years from conception onward, but now that the body has matured, it is function-structure that gives a truer insight into the clinical evaluations of the science of osteopathy as they apply to the patient.

The osteopathic physician has to learn to *feel* physiological functioning within, manifesting its ever-changing role in the structural economy of the patient. He needs to observe with his eyes, ears, and touch the differences between the normal and abnormal changes in function within any given area in any given specialty in osteopathy.[1]

I believe that the concept of structure-function in which we have a framework surrounded by tissues and in which structure determines function is certainly valid. The other side of the coin, in which we have a living mechanism in which function-structure is more dominant in the outward expression of life as we live it in our day-to-day health and disease patterns, is equally valid in terms of clinical analysis and understanding.

Developing Palpatory Skill

Now, for item number two, the art of developing a trained palpatory sense. Let us begin with the fact that you have an upper extremity, extending all the way from the shoulder girdle down through to the

1. W.G. Sutherland, *Contributions of Thought*, 2nd ed., pp. xvii–xviii.

fingertips. If we want to develop fingertip control over the structures we are examining and to expand our ability to learn to use it with greater understanding in determining either structure-function or function-structure, we're going to have to take into consideration the total upper extremity. So, anatomically, let us consider the total upper extremity—the scapula, clavicle, humerus, radius, ulna, eight carpal bones, five metacarpals, and all the phalanges. These are surrounded by muscles, ligaments, and tendon sheaths; are covered with skin; and all these tissues are thoroughly bathed by the fluids of the body. The upper extremity is also loaded with thousands of nerve endings, especially in the palmar surfaces of the fingertips, with nerves extending up through the deeper structures, up to the brachial plexus and the cervical and upper thoracic spine.

We have a superficial set of nerve endings for palpatory touch in the surface of the skin. We also have deeper proprioceptive fibers, the function of which is to allow us to determine the position of our hand or arm in its total relationship to where we have it hanging in space. In developing your palpatory sense of touch, you're going to use both the superficial sensory nerves for touch and the deeper proprioceptive fibers which are associated with all the muscles and ligaments from the fingertips all the way back up through the shoulder girdle.

As an exercise, pick up an ordinary ball in one hand. Feel the roundness of it with your hand, with the fingertips, with the palmar surface of the hand itself. Notice its texture and consistency. Here you are using the surface contact of your hand and the muscles of the hand to determine the qualities and texture of this ball you have picked up.

Now, add to this palpatory sense by bringing into play the proprioceptive fibers in the whole upper extremity, from the spinal cord and shoulder girdle down to the hand. Be conscious of the fact that you are feeling that ball with the whole extremity—not with just the hand contact alone—and immediately, you will note that you have an entirely different, far deeper appreciation of that same ball as compared with the experience of just observing with the hand contact alone.

Right now, I'm holding a package of cigarettes in my hand. It is a rectangular package filled with 20 cigarettes. But when I invoke the deeper sense of feeling with the total extremity, as I grasp the same package of cigarettes with no more pressure on it than I would if I were just holding it in my hand, I am conscious of the fact that I've added a sense of three-dimensionality to my feeling. I feel as if I'm feeling all through the package, rather than just holding onto the surface of the package. That is step number one—add the proprioceptive sense of feeling with the entire upper extremity and shoulder girdle to the object you are holding.

Step number two is to consider the total upper extremity and shoulder girdle as a lever, similar to a lever you would use in prying up a boulder. Here again you get the idea that instead of merely feeling with the end of the lever which is against the boulder, you're feeling that boulder with the total lever. Now, add a fulcrum point anywhere along that lever, and we have added a control point, a source of power. We can pull down on one end and immediately effect a change at the other end of the lever against that boulder so as to make it move.

I've used this same thought in trying to discuss "diagnostic touch," but I want to get away from that—I want to talk about function and structure. If I establish a fulcrum point and apply compression at that fulcrum point, creating a sense of power, I am affecting both ends of the lever. My shoulder girdle is at the upper end of the lever, and my hand contact is at the lower end. If I push my hand up against that boulder, I am going to apply power through to it and move the boulder. But if instead I apply compression at the fulcrum point and leave my hand contact quiet, I will be able to sense more in that boulder, without necessarily moving it, than I would if I did not have a fulcrum point somewhere along the length of the lever.

When I shift from feeling with just my superficial hand contact to feeling with my whole upper extremity, I feel a great deal more. If I apply a fulcrum point, I can feel even more because now I have a total lever with a fulcrum point. And then applying compression at the fulcrum point gives me a point of control to feel even deeper, with all the proprioceptive fibers, from one end of the lever to the other.

In summary, I have described three levels of sensory input which make available to you three levels of palpatory skill. These skills can be used to assess the function-structure or structure-function of the body. The first level is to feel with the palmar surface of the hand only, using the sense of touch in the superficial nerve fibers. The second level is to sense with the total proprioceptive sense of the entire upper extremity and shoulder girdle as you feel the object you are holding. The third level is to establish a fulcrum point along the line of the lever and sense with the total lever mechanism from the shoulder girdle on down, with the added emphasis of applying some degree of compression at the fulcrum point. When adding the compression, you are not necessarily raising your hand into the tissue but merely applying compression at the fulcrum point so as to bring in a still deeper layer of evaluation in the total picture. In this way, you get three different evaluations of the same object you are examining. You can try this on anybody or anything. You may use all three or any one of the three in examining any object you choose to place your hands on or work with.

13. CORRESPONDENCE:
WILLIAM G. SUTHERLAND, D.O.

*These are edited excerpts from letters written by Dr. Becker to William
G. Sutherland, D.O. Dr. Sutherland's responses, where available, are
included. Excerpts were selected for inclusion to show Dr. Becker's
early thinking and the development of his understanding through the
decade of his close association with Dr. Sutherland. Included at the end
is a letter from Dr. Becker's mother written upon the occasion of
Dr. Sutherland's death.*

December 22, 1949

The more I study Osteopathy, the more it seems to boil down to
a Highly Intelligent fluid surrounded and held in shape by fascial
membranes.

Allow the fascial strains to correct what might be present, allow
the fluid to resume its normal TIDAL mechanism, and all associated
pathologies in the muscle, skin, blood vessels or nerves will correct
themselves. "Bend to the oar" through the fascia, and "ride the TIDE
to the shore" by way of the fluid.

February 3, 1951

I need your help and advice. As you know, I became conscious of
the Master Fulcrum and talked to you about it in Des Moines. However, my understanding of it at that time was certainly in the embry-
onic stage, and I have been running into problems.[1]

1."Master Fulcrum" is a term that does not appear in any of Dr. Sutherland's published
writings, and the only appearance of it in Dr. Becker's work is in his correspondence
with Dr. Sutherland.

Before I go further, I think you will be interested in the enclosed drawings which the Russian artist has made of spirals within spirals within the human body. You have probably seen them. If not, here they are. It is a graphic way to express the function of whatever tissue he is trying to portray. The Master Fulcrum might almost be compared to a Master Spiral for the total mechanism, with hundreds of smaller ones for individual function.

Back to my problem. I find I cannot treat in the way I used to without overtreating the patient when I apply the Master Fulcrum approach. My present approach is to position the patient on the table with the feet against the footboard, gently lay my hands on the head with the parietal hold, initiate a little action in the cerebrospinal fluid Tide, and quiet myself to seek and obey orders from the Master Fulcrum. There are two steps I am beginning to believe aren't necessary even with that simple approach—one is placing the feet against the footboard and the other is to initiate the Tide. However, to continue, I find that any problem in the fascial, membranous, osseous, autonomic, or central nervous system—wherever in the body mechanism— seems to come to the forefront, and then it goes to work, unlocks its unphysiological factors for that day, and settles down to the short rhythmic fluctuation of an alternate lateral and AP [anteroposterior] fluctuation. If instead I use the approach I was taught by Dr. Anna Slocum, my patients spend the next few days with so much to handle, they are extremely uncomfortable.

There is far more to this Master Fulcrum approach than can be described or told about. I am conscious of being in the presence of the factor that makes us tick. Knowledge of what I am working with has created a sense of something so tremendous that all my sense of values is going to have to be revised in using the science of osteopathy. My philosophy says that the Master Fulcrum can do no wrong, that it will work for the best interest of the patient at all times. It has such potential that I sense but don't understand.

Well, that about expresses my problem as accurately as I am able at this point. A few words from you would be appreciated. Am I oversimplifying my approach? Can you give me a clue as to how to get a closer insight into that which I am working with? Am I heading down the main trail or am I sidetracking?

If this sounds confused, it's because it probably is. All I know is that my patients are making some nice progress. But I want to know *why* and *how*, in order to continue to render the service that should be given them.

February 8, 1951   *Response from Dr. Sutherland*

...Just how to help you with the problem is somewhat difficult. But, *the thought strikes me* on some area of the intellectual recording brain that you will answer that question yourself. In fact, inasmuch as you keep close to the Fulcrum, it will come to you. And: I KNOW that you keep close to the Fulcrum.

From my study window there is a lovely view overlooking the Ocean, and a lighthouse. So: "Light in the darkness, sailor, Day is at hand" etc.[2] It will reflect throughout your problem. I KNOW it.

February 14, 1951

The LIGHTHOUSE is reflecting:

A.T. Still, *Autobiography*, pg. 148, "...I am fully convinced that God, of the mind of nature, has proven His ability to plan (if plan be necessary) and to make or furnish laws of self, *without patterns,* for the myriads of forms of animated beings; and to thoroughly equip them for the duties of life, with their engines and batteries of motor force all in action." *Emphasis added by Dr. Becker.*

March 1, 1951

Have been getting a lot of reflections lately, and they seem to add up to sensible figures for a change. You know the quotation I sent you the other day–"...I am fully convinced that God, of the

---

2. This line is from a song about religious salvation entitled "Pull for the Shore," written by Phillip Paul Bliss in 1873.

mind of nature, has proven His ability to plan (if plan be necessary) and to make or furnish laws of self, without patterns for the myriads of forms of animated beings..."—seems to have unraveled a great mass of confused detail.

Some unravellings (correct me if I am wrong):

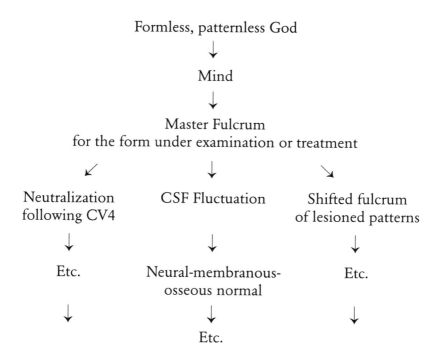

Formless, patternless God
↓
Mind
↓
Master Fulcrum
for the form under examination or treatment

Neutralization following CV4 — CSF Fluctuation — Shifted fulcrum of lesioned patterns

Etc. — Neural-membranous-osseous normal — Etc.

Etc.

All divisions under Master Fulcrum are but manifestations of the Master Fulcrum in action. A shifted fulcrum is not a cause of the lesioned pattern that is diagnosed. It is but a manifestation of the cause. The breakdown under each heading could go on indefinitely.

To take a given case as close to the Master Fulcrum as possible is to give it an opportunity to refold and unfold again as a pattern closer to that which is the Master Fulcrum.

August 28, 1951

Will, I have been having some mighty "uncanny" experiences. I sure do wish we could have another gabfest because it is hard to express them on paper. I am getting my signals from the stillness more and more, including the "all clear." When the signal comes, I check the physical mechanism and find the "boss" has come home.

Saw a young fellow the other day, 38 years old, with a history of constant illness for three years, including a decompensating mitral stenosis. Last week I treated him, and he went into a total extension type pattern that almost shut off his respiratory mechanism. He stayed in it for over 30 minutes. I could relieve him some by throwing the mechanism into flexion, but back he would go into extension when I eased up. I wasn't watching or obeying my signals as I should have because he would get so embarrassed for air he would get panicky. I finally let him go into extension and forced him right out the small end of the telescope. It only lasted five minutes, and he released the physical pattern and the "all clear" came shortly thereafter. When he sat up, he brought up a cupful of bloody sputum but slept like a baby that night and has been feeling good since. He could have released much sooner if I had reversed the telescope quicker. Live and learn.

September 12, 1951

Well, another gadget slipped behind the curtain.[3] I believe it was the last time that I wrote you that I was trying to find the main Tide of the ocean in my patient and bring it to a point of stillness. I did to the best of my ability and was getting results superior to previous efforts. Last night I took home your "Lighthouse Beams" for Ardath [Mrs. Becker] to read, and while she was reading them, I got to studying the Tide in the dictionary, in discussion with her, etc.[4] All of a sudden, the Tide slipped behind the curtain.

Just how many more gadgets are there in front of the curtain? Every time I see another one slip behind the curtain I think that might

---

3. For an explanation of the phrase "behind the curtain," see p. 240.
4. "The Lighthouse Beam" was the name of a brief series of newsletters Dr. Sutherland distributed to his teaching faculty. See W.G. Sutherland, *Contributions of Thought*, 2nd ed, p. 254.

be the last one, but am now willing to concede that there must be quite a pile left.

My next tour of investigation is to examine the full meaning of the Potency in your expression: the Potency of the Tide. As near as I can figure it now the Potency, the Intelligence, the Knowing and the Breath of Life are all the same thing. Their application is the Science of Knowing.

Examine the patient with the microscopic knowing of Dr. Still, find the lesion, put it in the spaces and watch it disappear into the void. It is all one operation, but if I have to describe it in steps, that is how I would do it.

Your "Lighthouse Beam" and Milwaukee talk were wonderful. You are bringing the osteopathic concept out in big bright letters that we can all begin to see and know. We are deeply grateful.

The Cartoonist has enclosed a series of five cartoons for your approval.

1. Breath of Life
   Knowing
   Intelligence
   Potency

2. Breath of Life
   Knowing
   Intelligence

3. Breath of Life
   Knowing

4. Breath of Life

5.

October 16, 1951

I am invited to speak to the New York Academy [of Osteopathy] on pathological physiology of the cervical spine including the cervicodorsal overlap and pretracheal drag. I would like to bring out Reciprocal Balanced Tension in normal and lesion patterns....

I thought I would build my presentation around three key statements I read in Carl McConnell's article on ventral technique to bring out the inherent Breath of Life of the living tissue. McConnell says, "It seems to be difficult for some students to grasp the osteopathic import of adjustment. They apparently forget that it rests upon the physiologic principle of self-adjustment." Again, "The real mystery of technic is centered in the life impulse, and in how little effort is required to normalize a region provided the application is precise." Again, "In clinical practice it is helpful to hold the view that the life impulse is not created (for it is of an eternal nature)."

December 20, 1951

Reflections from the "Lighthouse Beam": You have, I am sure, attended a symphony concert and observed the manner in which it was conducted. The Conductor mounts the podium, taps his baton, raises his arms in a moment of silence, brings them down and the symphonic piece is under way. It may be a most complicated score with the woodwinds sighing, the brasses blowing, and the multiple violins swinging and swaying in intricate patterns of crescendos, then pianissimos. The main theme may be carried by one group of instruments and then again by another. Intricate interweaving harmonics from the rest of the instruments, not concerned with the main theme, supplement the piece to give it richness. The description could be carried on and on by a musician. The orchestration usually terminates by bringing together all the instruments in a final blending, and as the last note dies away, there is a moment of silence again before the audience applauds their efforts.

You made a statement in your recorded lecture that has given me many moments of quiet contemplation: "...that still, small point between inhalation and exhalation." I don't recall the exact words, but the location was *between* flexion and extension, inhalation and exhalation, etc. The fulcrum point, you called it. Now it is fairly easy to visualize and *know* when you are at the top of the wave or the bottom of the trough as that can, with training, be felt through the senses. But that midway point is something else. I believe that I have found it and have been able to initiate such a starting point in my patients.

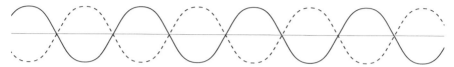

I submit the following observation to substantiate my claim. Bringing the patient to a point anywhere on the fulcrum line, as represented by the straight line in the illustration above, is similar to the conductor bringing the orchestra to the moment of silence before beginning the symphonic piece. Then the most intricate unfolding and refolding patterns of fluids, fascias, and tissue actions and reactions take place during the ensuing period, and finally it comes to a blending within the whole mechanism and terminates "in the fullness of the Tide." It was at this point that I have said to you that the "boss has come home and I can quit the treatment." All the activity takes place behind the curtain, and there is no need for interference. Some of the orchestrations are of a rather violent nature, and some are the loveliest sonatas ever heard. But all are initiated by that moment of stillness as the conductor raps his baton for attention. I believe that I am beginning to find that moment of silence which initiates the first movement.

Some corollary observations: This is going to render obsolete what I have believed until now, which is that there are four stages for the fluid mechanism: 1) organization of the fluid, 2) focusing of the fluid, 3) moment of stillness, and 4) balancing of new pattern. This mechanism is true for the fluid, fascias, ligaments, etc., but these are fulcrum points at the tops of the crests and the bottoms of the troughs and are merely some of the harmonics within the body of the symphonic selection.

That is it. Your comment and correction is eagerly awaited.

December 27, 1951   *Response from Dr. Sutherland*

Everything was *In Tune*, like a perfect fugue. Your "Boss" as the "Conductor" certainly "observed a moment of silence" wherein we recognized "Peace on Earth." In this reference you will find my "comment" for which you are "eagerly awaiting." The thought is *"greatly* to be appraised."

February 7, 1952

As usual, your most welcome comment to my letter opened about six more doors that I hadn't even considered. Have had many occasions since to "observe a moment of silence wherein we recognize Peace on Earth" in my patients. Needless to say, the subsequent manifestations far exceed my expectations. For which I thank you.

February 14, 1952

Some random thoughts from a rambling mind: I sure do like your expression the SeaAroundUs.[5]

One of the qualities of the Breath of Life is manifested as Knowing. The SeaAroundUs is one constant body of water with myriads of interchanging patterns in constant motion. The unifying Breath of Life is the automatic shifting suspension fulcrum through which the ever-changing patterns seek to balance each other. Knowledge of the Wholeness of the SeaAroundUs permits proper evaluation of the ever shifting, ever-changing patterns. These patterns are but tools. The cause lies within the Fulcrum.

The science of osteopathy is expressed through the Breath of Life as a Knowing of the Wholeness of the human body. The ever-changing patterns of fluid—including the chemical cerebrospinal fluid, membranes, fascias, osseous tissues and organized systems—interchange in countless changing patterns in response to the fulcrums within the

---

5. Dr. Sutherland had read and appreciated Rachel Carson's book, *The Sea Around Us* (1950).

body. The cerebrospinal fluid has a more important function in transmuting the Breath of Life of the SeaAroundUs into the qualities required by the chemical physical body. The body juices are the final expression of this transmutation process as they interchange in their myriads of motion patterns, always seeking balance.

The osteopathic physician as a mechanic of the Science of Knowing has the knowledge of the Wholeness of the patient before him. Therefore, because he can see the whole picture, he has the capacity to evaluate the component parts properly. For all that can be seen, heard, and felt on a sense level is but a tool and as a tool responds to the automatic shifting suspension fulcrums within the body. The Breath of Life is the one unifying factor for the total mechanism. The Breath of Life is *the* automatic shifting suspension fulcrum for the individual and serves to integrate the individual with the SeaAroundUs.

Perfect health is a balanced interchange between the body and the SeaAroundUs. The pattern of stress and strain can be brought back to health by "observing a moment of silence wherein we recognize Peace on Earth."

February 15, 1952

Ardath asks me to please interpret what I said yesterday, in terms she can understand, and to try to clean up the debris. So here goes:

SeaAroundUs: Light; One Eternal ever-present Light, Oneness.

Light or Oneness is the one constant Cause, Balance. It is manifested in electrical currents, tides, myriads of interchanging patterns in constant motion; all of these expressions centered by the unchanging Light, Potency, Cause. The Breath of Life is the individual spark of Light that centers the individual, and one of its qualities within the individual is manifested as Knowing. Knowledge of the Wholeness of the Light permits proper evaluation of the ever-shifting, ever-changing patterns. These patterns are but tools, manifested in motion; the cause lies within the Light, the Fulcrum.

The Breath of Life centers the individual. Utilizing the quality of Knowing, we as physicians have a Knowledge of the Wholeness of the human body. The ever-changing patterns of fluid—including the physical cerebrospinal fluid, membranes, fascias, osseous tissues and organized tissues—interchange in countless changing patterns in response to the Light within which knows only balance. The cerebrospinal fluid has a more important function in transmuting the Breath of Life or Light into the electrical and other qualities required by the chemical physical body. The body juices express the products of this transmutation process as they interchange in their myriads of motion patterns, ever seeking Balance.

The osteopathic physician as a mechanic of the Science of Knowing has the Knowledge of the Wholeness of the patient before him. Therefore, because he can see the whole picture, he has the capacity to evaluate the component parts properly. For all that can be seen, heard and felt on a sense level is but a tool and as a tool is responding to the physical automatic shifting suspension fulcrums within the body. The fulcrums in turn are centered by Light, Breath of Life, Potency, an unchanging Oneness that gives the mechanic, through Knowing, the complete and proper picture. The Breath of Life is the one unifying factor for the total mechanism.

Perfect health is a balanced interchange between the individual and the Light—physically, mentally, emotionally. Patterns of stress and strain (chemically, electrically, physically, etc.) in the individual can be brought back towards health by "observing a moment of silence wherein we recognize Peace on Earth," the Light, the Breath of Life. A Knowledge of Knowing permits the physician to do this through his Knowing.

Thus in both diagnosis and treatment, a physician's Knowing gives him an accurate picture of cause and remedy to reach that cause.

February 25, 1952   *Response from Dr. Sutherland*
You certainly have a grand way of interpretation that carries inspiration.

March 10, 1952
I have a case history that you might be interested in, and like [the

comic strip character] Dick Tracy, I would like to say, "Did you ever see anything like this?"

I was called to the Stevens Park Osteopathic Hospital last week to see a three-day-old baby who had been delivered by face presentation. He was under oxygen when I arrived and had been for 48 hours. He was a nine-pound boy and as blue as some of those dusky-blue bindings on our professional books. In addition, he had no grasping reflex in his left arm and hand, and the left leg and arm were as "blue as a whetstone." He had to be fed by eyedropper. His breathing was labored and obviously was only a pump working and not the normal breathing of a mechanism truly alive. The vault on the skull would rise and fall with each breath.

Examination showed a marked extension of the entire craniosacral mechanism, a marked compression of the entire left base of the skull, and marked strain around the occipital-atlantal area. He had some fluctuation pattern in the area of the cisterna magna, but it was mighty weak.

Treatment: I had the intern support the sacrum, and I supported the fluid mechanism of the cranium. It took several minutes to diagnose the strain and to elicit any activity of the mechanism wanting to do something about its problem. I then tried a little decompression of the condylar parts but soon quit that and went back to the basic idea of trying to hold the fluid content in a balanced position and letting it do the work. Within 20 minutes all lesions were corrected. I did have to go down and release the atlas individually, but the rest of the mechanism was free. All this time the intern was saying, "My gosh, did you feel that and did you see that?" The baby continued to stay cyanotic.

Excellent results to that moment, but the job was half done. I couldn't elicit that the battery had the right amount of "juice" in it. The physical battery was in pretty good shape, but the Breath of Life was not in full possession. I turned the baby on its side and gently placed two fingers on the occiput and two on the sacrum. In about five minutes, he reared back into an extension position and came forward again, and immediately the Breath of Life began to function and the sacrum and occiput got as warm as they should. The edema of the scalp began to leave, the breathing of the baby was that of one that was taking in oxygen and exchanging it properly, the vault ceased to rise and fall with each respiration, the child began to cry, the left hand started to open and close, and the cyanosis of the left hand lessened. The baby was still cyanotic, but that was a minor detail. The intern's eyes were popping.

They left the baby under oxygen for the next 18 hours (after all the hospital has to get the credit). The next morning, they put the baby to the mother's breast. The baby was pink and nice. His left side was acting normally, and he grabbed onto his mother's breast as if he hadn't had food for three days, which he probably hadn't. The doctor whose case it was never called me to acknowledge the change, but the intern kept in touch and said the baby had no more trouble.

The one important detail of the story is to be sure the Breath of Life is in full command before releasing the case for that particular treatment. I have carried this factor into all treatments since, and needless to say, I could write you all day, "Did you ever see anything like this?" It was worth all the work of the past eight years to be put in a position to render the service that was possible to that small child, and to the many others that I see in daily practice. We, in the osteopathic profession, are deeply grateful to you for the knowledge you have given us and for the method of presenting it to us.

March 20, 1952

You weren't kidding when you stated in "The Lighthouse Beam": *The main arena is the sea*; *the space between*; we visualize *the space between the grains of sand* and *know* that the solid rock is crumbling back into sandy grains; *the space between* the physiologic centers within the floor of the fourth ventricle.[6]

A membranous-articular strain or ligamentous-articular strain

---

6. W.G. Sutherland, *Contributions of Thought*, 2nd ed., p. 254.

suddenly releases its tension as a form of clay when it enters the spaces and takes on reciprocal tension that has Intent, Purpose, Meaning. In its new releasing patterns, it goes back to the position of the original strain and dissolves. Uncanny is no name for it. Outside the space, it is action and reaction in the physical sense, and charge and discharge in the electrical sense. In the spaces, it is a process of seeking Balance in the truest meaning of the word. 'Tis quite an experience to observe, and what a thrill!

March 21, 1952

Dr. Becker describes for Dr. Sutherland a visit from a colleague and then proceeds to write: ...He, too, had been hearing tales that I had gone off the deep end on this subject, or didn't you know that I was supposed to be off my rocker? But, by the last night he said, "I have been living too many years by stimulating a response and watching reactions in my patients and in my friends and in my living." Enough said.

April 28, 1952

The SeaAroundUs has been telling me some wonderful tales, and I thought I would consult with you as to their authenticity. For some reason or other my whole mess of cute little fulcrums all disappeared behind that curtain. The stage behind the curtain is going to get so full of gadgets there won't be room to move around in it. I got all worked up and enthusiastic about the spaces, and all of a sudden it didn't seem to have much importance anymore. But I do have something to talk about and my vocabulary is not satisfactory.

You say in your "Lighthouse Beam" that "the main arena is the sea," and you quote Rachel Carson, "There is no drop of water in the ocean, not even in the deepest parts of the abyss, that does not *know* and respond to the mysterious forces that *create the tide.*"[7]

The SeaAroundUs is perceptible in every patient and in every

---

7. R. Carson, *The Sea Around Us*, 1950; emphasis added by Dr. Becker.

event of life. It is real and it can be known. The resulting tide can be felt by knowing fingers and knowing senses. The knowledge of it and its potency, as one's fingers contact firmly but gently, permits the operator to realize that here is the source of the mysterious forces that create the tide. What is the source? I don't know. I, as the operator, only know that if I keep my vision upon the sea and not upon the resulting tides, currents, eddies and waves, that I can "bend to the oar, sailor, and ride the tide to the shore."[8]

Why is an operator necessary? That is the question that has caused me no end of trouble. You and Adah [Mrs. Sutherland] and I sat together in a hotel room one night in Milwaukee, and the SeaAroundUs did its work. I have seen it work on others without the use of the operator's hands. I suppose the answer lies in the fact that this is primarily a sense world we live in, and the operator, with his contacts, is like the skipper of the boat. His steady hand, his knowledge of the elements around the situation, and his guiding influence help to see that the voyage is more comfortable, and when the trip is finished, he knows that all is secure for that trip upon the sea. An operator is necessary, yes, in this electrical universe, but he should know and use "the mysterious forces that create the tide" to do the work in treating each case. Therefore, let us call this mysterious force the Breath of Life and hold a true course towards it.

May 8, 1952

Your description of the function of the pineal gland as a reflector in function, comparable to the moon's effect on the tides of the ocean, was very appealing to me. As a result I have a new diagram for your consideration:

---

8. This phrase refers to a song about religious salvation entitled "Pull for the Shore," written by Phillip Paul Bliss in 1873. A part of the refrain is as follows: "Pull for the shore, sailor...Heed not the rolling waves, but bend to the oar. Safe in the life boat, sailor, cling to self no more."

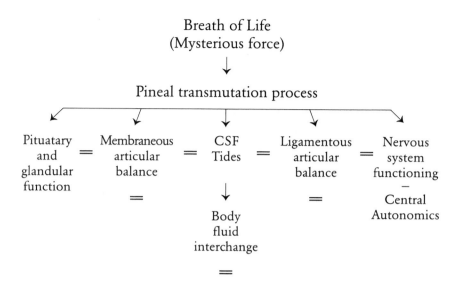

Everything below the transmutation process is in constant inter-changing reciprocal tension balance—electrically, biochemically, mechanically—charge and discharge—automatic shifting suspension fulcrums of expression of function as a result of power from the Breath of Life.

All is in the SeaAroundUs, and we all have the same SeaAroundUs in constant operation, and motivated by the same Breath of Life.

'Tis a great universe. I hope to someday know something about it.

August 31, 1952

My talk for the Colorado state meeting, "Added Tools in Osteopathic Diagnosis," is going to be just that. It makes me provoked when you ask most of the osteopathic physicians you meet nowadays, "What is osteopathy?" "Why, it is a treatment, of course," comes the answer. A. T. Still ought to be a whirling dervish, rolling over in his grave. I read [a recent textbook on] "principles of osteopathy" from cover to cover and that is an example. For the work as it is presented and for the emphasis on structural therapeutics it gets an "A" for effort and work, but for the original principles as taught by Still and by you and by my dad [Arthur D. Becker, D.O.] and by Carl

McConnell and by a lot of the men who were close to Still, the book
is a sad piece of work. All of which is a prelude to the fact that in
Colorado I hope to call to their attention that Still said "explore this
area," "we must hunt," "what is the cause?" etc. and then try to point
out some of the principles of the body's fascia and fluid mechanism
in normal and pathological physiology.

I found the notebook that Dad used in teaching principles the
other day and perused it carefully. The thing that strikes you is the
fact that he covers the subject he is discussing thoroughly and in detail, but nevertheless, there is a totality about it that indicates he has
the whole problem at his finger tips. His approach had the total effect
of indicating: What is wrong here in this case before you? Where is
the cause? What is the diagnosis? Why is this area normal and that
one a pattern of dysfunction? Diagnosis, diagnosis of cause. Treatment is there, but the emphasis is on why is *this* patient sick?

I may be wrong, but I think this is closer to what Still was thinking
about rather than "structural therapeutics." Right or wrong?

Another thought. In reading up about fascia for the Colorado talk,
I came upon the statement in Still's *Philosophy of Osteopathy*, "When
you deal with the fascia you deal and do business with the branch
office of the brain, and under the general corporation law, the same
as the brain itself, and why not treat it with the same degree of respect?" [p. 167]. That statement has caused me to study it many times.
With the peculiar behavior of the fascia and the ligaments in taking
them to the fulcrum point of their stress pattern, and watching the
tissue take the final smoothing analytical pattern inherent within that
pattern and proceeding to its own inherent correction within your
hands while you sit there and watch it, it makes one think the brain is
within your hands and that fascia does have the capacity to operate
independently of muscle, organ, bone, or whatever it contains. This
would be one interpretation of the "extension of the brain" idea. But
then again, fascia and all other containers of the body must obey the
position of the automatic shifting fulcrum within the individual mechanism or portion of the body, and the changes you feel while initiating

the inherent healing correction of the body and the act of correction itself are the dynamic effects taking place because "Cause" has been reached and the shifting fulcrum is correcting the mechanism. With this interpretation, brain and fascia are one and the same, but both are tools for use in the dynamics of physiological functioning.

I have another experience to tell you about. It is one that I hope you will discuss in Denver. There are lesions, if you can call them that, of the CSF tide. Will your talk on "manual alteration in the rate, direction and amplitude of the CSF" cover some of this material? By lesions I mean this: After I have heard the symptomatology, and the structural strains have been diagnosed to explain those symptoms, I sit down at the head and use a vault approach (though frankly any approach is just a matter of contact). One is conscious of the fact that in the total unit that represents that individual a new expression of the tide is working to maintain the total pattern that exists. The expression one senses is but an effect, but it is there. Furthermore, it is diagnosable and very interestingly diagnostic. In some it is a sense of total drag, in some it is a sense of nervous irritability expressing itself within the person, but still they are fatigued to a point of total inefficiency. In some it gives the impression the total problem is in the structural field and in others in the chemical field and in others in the endocrine field. Many impressions are present and thoroughly interesting to observe. I call it "lesion of the tide" because one senses that the total fulcrum of the life stream feeding that individual is at variance with the normal tide.

After diagnosis is observed, attention to it—the normal tide, the total fulcrum, the Master Fulcrum, the Breath of Life or whatever you care to call it—results in changes that cannot be described. Needless to say, my results the past few months have been "different" to put it mildly.

After reading this hodgepodge, I can see Ardath saying, "But why write all that? It surely could be expressed a lot more simply."

September 5, 1952 *Response from Dr. Sutherland*

...Wish we were going to the state meeting in Colorado in order to hear your presentation that will surely *ring* with early reflections by such real Doctors of Osteopathy, like A.D. Becker and E.C. Pickler, with whom I have memories of pleasant association in the state of Minnesota, and likewise the real article like McConnell with whom it was my privilege, with a few others, to receive private instruction. Keep the bells ringing with early refections. "Why is *this* patient sick?" is right. These early D.O.'s were thinkers, and they were "thinking osteopathy" *with* Doctor Still.

It is rather difficult to tell just what I may have to say about the subject assigned: "Manual alteration of rate, direction and amplitude of the CSF." Some of the thoughts in my mind might be better left unsaid. It is always easy to talk unintelligently about a subject which we know so little about.

But what I may say need not affect your presentation of your subject assigned. The "fluid water" is certainly *deep*. The "fluid-drive" on the car was patterned after the fluctuation of the cerebrospinal fluid, and we know that in man's pattern there can be lesions. Just how the terminology fits into the body mechanism, or can be explained to others, becomes difficult.

At any rate, "manual alteration of the rate, direction and amplitude of the CSF" may be summed up briefly as: An expression of nonincisive surgical skill to secure balance in the laws attributed to the fluid mechanism, or balance in "the laws not framed by the human hand."[9]

October 13, 1952

I thought you might be interested in some follow-up on the themes we talked about in Denver and their application during these few days back at home. Well, they work—they work one hundred percent of the time.

Needless to say, my gratitude to you folks [Will and Adah Sutherland] goes beyond words. Fortunately, I think you know how deeply we feel on this subject, so let it suffice to say that Ardath and I thank you.

---

9. "I do not claim to be the author of this science of Osteopathy. No human hand framed its laws..." (A.T. Still, *Autobiography*, p. 302).

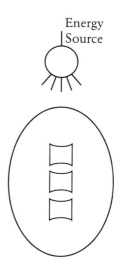

One of the things that clung to my reflections about our discussions was the fact that you, Will, disconnected the energy source on my little figure of a body of fluid surrounded by a membrane and containing an osseous mechanism. How right you are. We are in relation to the whole universe and respond or reflect as positive and negative spirals in relation to the whole—not to the limited mechanism within our skins. As Still puts it, "...the all-knowing Architect has cut and numbered each part to fit its place and discharge its duties in every building in animal form, while the suns, stars, moons, and comets *all obey the one eternal law of life and motion.*"[10]

To connect this up to my first week back, my habit patterns wanted to find the relation of the so-called lesion to other patterns *within* the body. The relationship was there but not in a primary sense. I kept at it and insisted my mechanism get out of the way, and pretty soon I found I was finding the relationship of the pattern under treatment to the whole, and as it would slip into the total understanding, I found that I needed new tools with which to appraise what was going on. There is where "The Lighthouse Beam" came in handy.[11] The proprioceptive touch we teach the students is not sufficient to use in the "spaces." The operator's as well as the patient's mechanism disappears behind the curtain.[12] As I told you in Denver one day, "The whole darn works has disappeared." I found out I wasn't kidding. It looks as if the old song, "Me and My Shadow," is all wrong. Only the shadow exists, and it is only a reflection in constant motion.

This could go on and confuse you more, but I will stop for now and will send more later as things work out. It is as if we were working with reality and seeing the reasons why for the first time in our professional career. I am looking forward to more time with you.

---

10. A.T. Still, *Autobiography*, p. 149; emphasis added by Dr. Becker.
11. W.G. Sutherland, *Contributions of Thought*, 2nd ed., p. 254.
12. For an explanation of the phrase "behind the curtain," see p. 240.

December 8, 1952

...Here's an idea for my upcoming talk on the fascias of the cardiac and circulatory systems: The circulatory system is essentially a floating mechanism, from heart to capillary and return, supported by a fascial framework that must be free to permit normal action. The pericardium is supported from the styloid processes above and the central tendon of the diaphragm below, and from ligamentous processes from the manubrium and the xiphoid process. It floats! From that beginning, it goes on and on.

I just found out recently what an essentially lonely man you may have been for these many years, Will. You have been sitting with Still, McConnell and others at the hub, or fulcrum, if you please, and watched the wheels turn, the sand scrape, and the friction develop between and among those of us who thought we were heading towards the fulcrum while we were actually highly intrigued by the bright lights and action of the periphery. I know that to be true, and how did and do you have the patience to see so much fumbling and still keep your poise? I say this because I have been very lightly exposed to a small portion of that loneliness in recent weeks when I tried to expose a supposedly interested cranial group to some of the material that was taught at Denver. Tom Schooley's talk went over their heads like a cloud at night. It was never seen, thanks probably to my poor presentation. What would they not see if they were exposed to some of the material you gave me?

BUT, my patients have been exposed to this greater knowing through the application of its principles to the best of my knowledge, and the results have been those that you talk about. "Wait until you see some of the uncanny results in your practice," said Dr. Sutherland, and he was right. The SeaAroundUs is present in all of us and at all times, and *it* is welling up in every case and manifesting a magnitude equal to that of the heavens. Yes, you have been lonely but 'tis a marvel to me that you have been able to find as many words to describe the fulcrum and its manifestations as you have and are doing so well. Keep it up. We love it.

January 22, 1953

The latest integration program as a result of the discussions we had (and didn't have) in Kirksville emerges from the spaces. Enclosed is a chart to illustrate what I hope I can put into words.

The Breath of Life, God, is a symbol of perfection, of balance. Balance is the point at which ebb and flow equalize in rhythmic balanced interchange in dynamic capacity, or maybe balance is a *space* not a point where rhythmic balanced interchange takes place. I'll take the latter view—it just occurred to me.

The upper chart with its three spaces to represent the doctor, patient, and God all represent the same Breath of Life in rhythmic balanced interchange. Since the three are One, I drew it as One for the second chart.

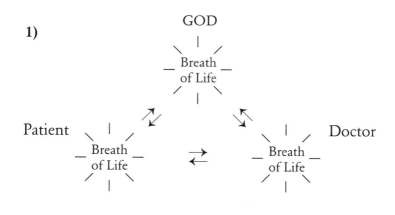

Out of the One, God, Breath of Life, is the outpicturing of spirals, centered by the Breath of Life, for the perfect expression of rhythmic balanced interchange.

Since all material manifestations—man, environment, and his relationship to his fellow men—are centered by the same Breath of Life, bringing all components of his life to this center space, the Breath of Life, permits a new Balance, designed for perfection, to manifest itself.

Within each individual and his environment is the capacity to center himself in this common center, or, if it be necessary for him to seek help through others (the physician), it is within the capacity of the physician to center the patient, for it is the same Breath of Life that centers all life.

Since the Breath of Life is the same as the Space that shapes the universe, only a more perfect, dynamic Balance can manifest itself as the patient is brought into rhythmic balanced interchange with the Breath of Life.

The Breath of Life supplies laws that create the pattern and the energy in the form of ebb and flow to express the pattern. The pattern and its material energy-wave manifestations are as multitudinous as the infinite. All come from and are returned to the same Breath of Life.

Knowledge of what laws and patterns exist is in the spaces, and the capacity to change those laws and patterns to express a more rhythmic balanced pattern is in the same "space."

Yes, Will, your "spaces" and Breath of Life are POTENCY in practice, in knowledge, and available for instant use NOW.

The same old story. I hope I said it more clearly.

January 23, 1953

P.S. To the letter of yesterday. Ardath, bless her, says it can be written better to explain the Breath of Life and how it operates. So-o-o-o, here goes:

All our love to you,

Rollin and Ardath

P.P.S. What POTENCY the FULCRUM has with a SPACE over which to operate!

P.P.P.S. There aren't any limitations in the explanation above.

March 27, 1953

...holding fast to the Head, from whom the whole body, nourished and knit together through its joints and ligaments, grows with a growth that is from God.

Colossians 2:19 (Revised Standard Version)

I have been meaning to write you for a long time and express my feelings for the way you have guided the program of the Science of Osteopathy through Osteopathy in the Cranial Field. Working through the Head, through the trolley wire, Will has had very little to say about the programming, but Will, nevertheless, has done a beautiful job manifesting the job to be done.

You are Listening and you hear. You are being Directed and you demonstrate the results. You are Aware and your awareness is reflected through your work. The reflections have spread to hundreds of us and to thousands of people whom we serve.

You had no choice—the Breath of Life gave you the job and you responded and the job is continuing to unfold.

For all this we are thankful to you, grateful to you, and above all, we love you.

April 2, 1953 *Response from Dr. Sutherland*

...Thank you for the quotation from Colossians 2:19. And, most of all, greatest gratitude for your wonderful love.

April 25, 1953

Listen to the song of a discouraged man, and when you have read it, set a match to it and forget it.

First for my personal troubles. The time Dr. —— treated me in Des Moines in 1950, I went through five months of hades, and finally the load lifted physically and mentally and I was free to float again. Again in Kirksville this January, she treated me and I have had constant trouble with my sacral mechanics since, and though it hasn't put me into the depressed state I was in before for five months, I have not been comfortable. The only relief I get is when I take time out and say, "Be still." It helps for a time. The other time I received some relief was when Sam Hitch gave me a treatment, and even then he couldn't budge it or see results in the patterns until I relinquished myself to the spaces and stayed there to the best of my ability. I have had similar experiences in using her approach on patients, in that there are plenty of fireworks but no real peace in the problem afterwards.

Next I have a million questions and not a decent answer in the bunch. The routine methods of diagnosis prescribed by our modern osteopathic friends and modern medical science are all so gross and full of peripheral information that it has little meaning as to the real pattern within the patient. The same applies to a careful osteopathic structural examination, including the best craniosacral findings I can make. It still does not explain the patterns I find. Combining the two methods adds more confusion and information. The interesting thing to me is that I find "fulcrums"—focuses of activity around which a person operates—and a multiple change of tissue patterns, fluid fluctuations, etc., accompanying the focus or fulcrum, but there must be a time element in those patterns that I cannot understand. An example: A patient needs treatment, and I sense or am aware of a "fulcrum" off to the right. Going through the fulcrum to the Stillness, after a time, like sliding down a greased pole, the whole pattern moves to a centralized mechanism, without pattern, and the whole works clears up for a time. Then in a few days or weeks, the process must be repeated. Why? Why? Why?

If I attempt to cling to modern diagnostic measures, I am as futile in understanding my patient as are my colleagues. If I attempt to go to the Stillness and listen, fulcrums and patterns appear, but they do so in a terminology that can't be found in the books and apparently in a way that I fail to understand or comprehend with my sense of touch or with the physical thoughts that we call thinking. Neither suffice to explain, Why is this patient this way? In what way will they react to the attempt to unlock the pattern we find? Nor is there a prognostic indication of what is to come in the days ahead for that patient. Why? Why? Why?

I just saw a patient today who has a wicked pattern causing sciatica in the left leg, potentially a herniated disc. I have diagnosed and treated her 16 times in the past two years. She has been free of symptoms for the past six months, but she still has the pattern of stress in the left sacral area and a fulcrum of activity when we go to the spaces and get out of the road. Still she is free of symptoms. Why does not the pattern dissolve? Am I slipping on my local diagnosis? Should I treat locally? If I do, she gets poor results, but if I treat her through the Breath of Life, she does well symptomatically but the apparent pattern remains. Why?

Another woman gives a serious history of a frontal concussion seven years ago and has been having a nervous breakdown for the past year. Her doctor says she has a hysterical problem, problems with her second husband, etc.—the usual misinformation we get through conventional approaches. She has made rather a remarkable response to the Breath of Life, *but* each time she is treated, there is an erratic, shifted, shifting fulcrum that doesn't want to come home to the Boss. What is the time element that seems to be present in this problem? Why doesn't it come home and stay home? It did for three weeks; then went out of focus and stays there. Why? Why? Why?

So it goes in all the work I am doing. I feel like the preacher in the Bible, "All vanity and much striving after wind." The patients are happy, my business is on the increase, and my colleagues think I am nuts— but still call me in to diagnose their more difficult cases, and then I have a hell of a time writing the findings in terms they will understand. Terminology doesn't explain my findings. My "cranial" colleagues think I am wonderful. If they only knew the confusion I am in, they would change their opinion.

I see so much to learn. I see so much in modern diagnostic methods and findings I have to unlearn. I cannot coordinate the findings of the laboratory with the living mechanism under my observation. And I can no longer trust either my physical thoughts about their problems or gather enough information through my touch to satisfy the multiple patterns I know are present. Furthermore, I have not adequately learned the art of LISTENING and understanding for that which I know must be the right knowledge I should be receiving.

If I treat for best results, the patient goes to the Breath of Life and a new pattern comes out, NOW. I did not understand the old one very well, and the new one is incomprehensible in making future plans for treatment. In other words, all the physical attributes, including thought, do not work in using the Breath of Life. Where then is the answer?

In spite of our difficulties, we LOVE you, Adah and Wullie [one of Dr. Sutherland's nicknames], and may the best continue for you. Like I said: Get your match out!

May 6, 1953

I have been waiting to write until I felt that I could do so without having to later retract some of my thoughts. As you well suspected, much physical material, including the physical side of patterns and fulcrums, was doing a good job of sliding behind that old curtain.[13] Interestingly enough, to me at least, is their availability to meet the needs of given situations when called upon by the Boss, the Breath of Life, and then they quietly go behind the curtain again.

Personally, my physical problems have melted also, and all is going well.

More than ever I realize that the one reality, the Breath of Life, is an ever-living present NOW, and ALL revolves, manifests, comes forward, retreats, and expresses itself in the Breath of Life.

Many of the things that I observe and talk about to you when we are together take a few months to make themselves KNOWN to me, but they finally do and am I happy about it.

The view is much clearer and is so much more enjoyable when one doesn't have to carry so many parcels in their arms. Thank you, dear curtain. When one is working with the Breath of Life, there is no need for all that stuff that has gone behind the curtain. "May that curtain stay shut," I believe I have heard you say. I agree. The same is true for all of living and at all times.

_____

13. For an explanation of the phrase "behind the curtain" see p. 240.

June 25, 1953

This is a letter that is long overdue, and 'tis a pleasure to have the time to write it. The heart of your teaching, the Breath of Life, is manifesting its Potency hour after hour, day after day in a way that cannot be described. I am developing a deeper understanding of the Fulcrum with each passing day and can almost answer some of those questions I have thrown at you. I have added a few dozen more to take their place, and I am deeply disappointed that you will not be at Denver to listen to my prattling. I am going to discuss a point or two now as I see it and ask for comment, if you choose to give it.

A case in question: A lady was subjected to a twisting injury, falling between the front and back seats of a car in an automobile accident 15 years ago. She was hospitalized and casted and treated orthopedically for six months and finally went back to her occupation as a dancer. However, she continued to have enough trouble with her lumbar area to keep her going to doctors off and on for years. Three years ago she married a millionaire, and since then she has seen ten orthopedic specialists from coast to coast who have failed to explain her low back pain and the sense of insecurity she feels in that area. Many braces and many exercises have failed to have any particular influence.

My impression is that she is operating from a fulcrum, if you can call it that, that is about two feet anterior to her physical anatomy and located in space opposite her lumbar area. "Now that is a fine diagnosis, Doctor," says any intelligent scientific doctor. "Just what the hell do you mean?" Nevertheless, I am simply reporting what I observed as the Still Point came to a Pause-Rest. She reports immediate relief after a treatment and is encouraged for the first time that maybe something can be done for her.

Comment: The Breath of Life operates in the eternal NOW. The lady is manifesting an induced fulcrum of many years' duration, and the symptoms are the physical pattern permitted by this fulcrum in the now as a result of the gradual molding of physiological functioning to meet the fulcrum. I expressed it to her that I was treating the "shock" that occurred 15 years ago. When the Breath of Life can resolve or dissolve the induced fulcrum, she will return to the patternless form she had before, and the composite symptom form will disappear.

Damn words. They don't say what I want to say. I believe we live most freely in a patternless expression, endowed and maintained by a Breath of Life. Occasionally, we have other patterns imposed upon our well-being, and as long as they are in operation, we mold to fit them. The energy of their expression, whether it be disease or stress, comes from the same source, but it is not in balance with what God would like for us to have. Bringing these induced patterns into the Hands of God, the Breath of Life, permits His patternless expression to again manifest itself. The time element is of no importance as far as the Breath of Life is concerned. The physical, electrical manifestation may take time to unfold and refold according to our sense world, but the heart of the reality is the Breath of Life.

According to this wording, then, the lady in question will manifest "well-being" when the patternless form has and can be permitted to manifest itself. If this be true, what a wealth of reevaluation we must make in our thinking to interpret the present classification of disease and stress. If this be true, the reality is in the space and the unseen, and all the material that has been going behind the curtain, including electrical thinking, is only a transient blending of the moment and the unreal part of life. That is enough. Excuse the wordiness.

I think it most kind of you to let us fledglings play and run the courses. This is one fledgling that likes to have the Sun present and shining to stretch his wings in. There is less chance of error and running into obstacles and wrong teaching in the sunshine. You are a brave man to let us do it. It will slow down the quality of teaching considerably to not have you there. We are too materialistic in our approach and place too much emphasis on the stuff I have so vigorously been trying to get behind the curtain. It's not that we don't try to do the best we can—we just haven't learned to use our wings well enough yet.

July 16, 1953

I have some observations to make. I am not attempting to define anything, but am trying to record impressions I am currently observing. Your observation, "A mechanic in the science of KNOWING," on the long-playing record at first had the meaning for me that one should be able to record functional positions of fulcrums, patterns, etc., but I find now those are only the end results. "A mechanic in the science of KNOWING" is able to perceive the TIDE in operation—at least, that seems to be my impression the past few days. If KNOWING and TIDE are synonymous, then, as these patients come to me for observation, diagnosis, and treatment, and I am aware of an underlying quality of activity taking place beyond the fulcrums and patterns, at times during their stay in the office, momentary periods of STILLNESS occur depending on the problem, and in a few minutes the material picture changes considerably and always towards freedom.

The important point I am trying to state is that this underlying TIDE is universal, without definition, and has no real connection to the problems. Like the glass house you described in Kirksville, "The Breath of Life or TIDE does not touch the house but lights it up by reflecting through and through."

It is sufficient to observe the TIDE at work—that is the reality. What is to be done takes place, for the material products are but a reflection of their Source. The complex products of the medical science must obey the mandates of the TIDE, and the Intelligence to understand the complex products of the material manifestation is one of the rewards of the TIDE.

Enough, enough! It is possible to perceive the TIDE? It is permissible to place full reliance on the TIDE for diagnosis and treatment? The TIDE will deliver the highest quality of healing art available to man in his walk about on Earth?

August 11, 1953

The rather enthusiastic card I sent you July 31st—"What a Fulcrum! Wow!"—was sent on the spur of the moment and probably will express better the sentiments I wish to say than the present epistle.

Up until July 31st, there have been many times that, in the course of diagnosis and treatment, I have been led by the Tide to the Breath of Life—to that moment of stillness when the whole works is closer to our Maker than breathing. On July 31st and since, apparently at will, we start at the Breath of Life, from a still point, and radiate outward to unfold the whole pattern. On the one side we come from the periphery to the center, and on the other side we start from the center and go out. Does this make sense?

Ardath reported that she felt as though she were "fluid throughout." Another patient, who is very attuned, reported that once during a previous treatment, she felt worked from the outside in and came to a point in which she was closer to the Maker than breathing. This happened just once in many treatments given. Following July 31st, with her next treatment it happened again, and she reports it started from within and unfolded. By the way, this all began after I had been doing some serious meditating on, "What was all this about?"

I have formed other impressions since this has happened and would like to expound a little bit on them. I get the impression that bent twigs are being modified as I never saw them modified before.[14] I get an impression of the totality of the whole mechanism and the importance of the so-called restrictions within that mechanism, and yet these pale in their significance when one sees the Potency, the Power, the tremendous outpicturing that is unfolding from within the Fulcrum outward.

I get this impression: For each star in the firmament, there is a Fulcrum for it that keeps it in its place, that strives for an orderly expression of its spot in the universe. Similarly, each of us has a Fulcrum that expresses the normal, the rightness, the total capacity for functioning within our sphere of the universe. Note: I do not place

---

14. The term "bent twig" refers to the saying, "As the twig is bent so is the tree inclined." Dr. Sutherland used this phrase to refer to the effects that traumas sustained in birth and the developmental process can have.

this Fulcrum in any one location, in any relation to any set tissue relationship. It is present and is the Breath of Life for that individual. I now get the impression that as this Breath of Life is tapped, it supersedes all patterns, physical fulcrums, etc., and out of it unfolds or is transmuted the directions for the ideal pattern to be expressed in the total structure. All treatment that is given locally that is directed towards this master Fulcrum is an automatic transmutation towards the best that is available.

Interestingly enough, despite the power that is immediately expressed in the tissues during treatment and the changes that are taking place, the patient is much more comfortable and has little or no reactions to treatment compared to the reactions when we started at the periphery and came in on the problem.

I have been having my difficulties since this all began, wondering, Where am I now? With first things first and the ideal that is wanting to be expressed by the Breath of Life from the Fulcrum outward—shifts in fulcrums, patterns of stress and strain, patterns of disease or pathology just don't have the same importance or the same interpretation they did have. They are not what the Boss wants, and He goes about bringing in the normal NOW. Orthodox physiological understanding according to our noted authorities does not fit that which is unfolding within this patient.

Another difficulty: My previous concepts do not fit the things that are happening. My so-called knowledge of the principles involved are being modified, or will have to be, to appreciate what is going on.

Does all this make sense, or am I crazy?

Your Breath of Life is a *living* principle, and it can be called upon at will to create within this patient an outfolding of a normal physiological pattern in a normal anatomical mechanism. That is primary. The stresses and strains, the unphysiological pathology that is being expressed, are being superseded or transmuted into the normal—the stresses, etc., are not changing to the normal, the normal is replacing the trouble. I get the impression that the Potency released from the Breath of Life is transmuted into the cerebrospinal fluid, which in turn is activating the primary respiratory mechanism, which in turn is modifying the secondary mechanisms, etc. I am not being arbitrary in breaking this down. It is all one smooth expression of the Breath of Life and its manifestation into being in the physical levels.

What do you think of this scrabble? 'Tis sure fun to know and to use, and the nice thing about it is that the Breath of Life seems to be in complete charge of the whole process. I sure hope so. I'd hate to make some of the changes I see take place as fast as this inherent Potency changes them.

December 23, 1953

...P.S. There seems to be a universal pulse beat or fluctuation that follows the still point and has no relation to the physical fluid or fascial-ligamentous mechanism. It seems to be the same rate in all people, including children, and can be perceived before the "Still Point" but is more so after the Boss has spoken. You wouldn't want to confirm or deny a statement like that, would you?

December 27, 1953 *Response from Dr. Sutherland*

Thanks for the fine Christmas letter. No "confirmation" or "denial" to the postscript other than you are usually right.

February 3, 1954

...I dropped you a note saying the Boss was reorganizing my material for me. I started to say I was reorganizing some material about the Boss, but I see the Boss has stated it correctly. He reorganized it for me, and I have very little to report.

Much can be done for most problems provided several factors are considered: First, the normal must be known, and the normal includes a knowledge of the Boss and His desire for the normal to express itself. But what is normal? Something that A. T. Still suggested as, "...that God, of the mind of nature, has proven His ability to plan (if plan be necessary) and to make or furnish laws of self, without patterns, for the myriads of forms of animated beings; and to thoroughly equip them for the duties of life, with their engines and batteries of motor force all in action. Each part is fully armed for duty, empowered to select and appropriate to itself from the great laboratory of nature such forces as are needed to enable it to discharge the duties peculiar to its office in the economy of life."[15] That is quite an assignment—to be a being wholly capable of living and responding as described in that paragraph and to be in the constant position of being without plan or pattern, ever ready to select and appropriate to itself, etc. Yet it is also possible that under each bent twig we see, such a being exists.

Next, one needs knowledge of the physical nature so as to know each part and how it is constructed and how it fits. The abnormal, and that is highly speculative, is only an area that is doing the best it can under the circumstances. It can be observed objectively and assessed along with other information. It is interesting to observe some of the patterns that express themselves. Today I had one that manifested effects in the mental, emotional, and physical arenas, yet when the Boss stepped in, the whole process was transmuted, not dissolved, transmuted towards the normal.

Lastly (for this particular ramble of ideas), there is the question of why these patterns suddenly or chronically tend to manifest? I am not in a position to discuss this—I don't know. But I do know that in the transmutation process, as the Boss steps into the Fulcrum, there is a great deal more that goes on than a mere loss of a pattern of dysfunction. There is a Rebirth, a Regeneration of physical, mental, and emotional structure. To me it is like the world we were talking about in Denver, the world of total capacity for full constant functioning. It is quiet, serene, eternal, and can be measured objectively and subjectively. Just ask the patient. He feels like a "new person." And why not? He is.

---

15. A.T. Still, *Autobiography*, p. 148–49.

March 29, 1954

This note is to report a significant change in my application of the science of osteopathy. The thing that brought it to my attention has been "cranial" colleagues I have dealt with lately. We have had interactions, and I find I cannot understand them clearly anymore, as if I ever could.

It dawneth on me that I now evaluate my cases by searching for the quantity and quality of Light within them, and through that same Breath of Life, there is released a problem that has reflected physically, mentally, emotionally or in some combination thereof. In talking and working on these other D.O.'s, it is limiting to decide what pattern or shift of membranous or ligamentous articular mechanisms, when it is obvious that the Breath of Life is not manifesting its full potency, and why not go to it to allow physiological functioning to manifest its unerring potency?

A case or two to illustrate. 1) A 26-year-old woman, married five years, heavy vaginal discharge—painful and irritating for four years. Three treatments to correct a disturbed Breath of Life in the pelvic region and it is gone. Only one time did I use the pelvic lift. All three times I was at the sacrum observing the Breath of Life in the pelvic region come back to full strength in potency. 2) A woman who was half crazy and ready to be taken for shock treatment was brought in. It was obvious she was anchored at the sacrum. Five minutes later it released, and no trouble since. She had been this way for six months following a miscarriage. 3) A chronic case of depression—a withering field that had had ten electric shock treatments was brought back within a few weeks to essentially normal.

One outstanding failure: A 26-year-old woman whose only physical finding on thorough general physical examination is an extremely low-voltage wave on the electroencephalograph. She has been loyal in coming to me once a week for almost two years. She gives a history of two severe concussions, but outside of a deliberate miscarriage a few years ago, her history is negative. I have not been able to make one single impression on her problem through any and all approaches I can think of. I am baffled.

Even with that one lack of success and the usual number of problem cases we are always seeing, it is of interest to me that in using the Breath of Life primarily–working with and through it primarily–much, if not all, of the physical analysis as to what has slipped where and why has faded and disappeared, and my enthusiasm based on the results that have been attained has never been so high. It is most limiting to try to explain this to smart men like the colleagues I referred to when it is obvious that they are doing excellent work. But they are confused when I fail to use the mechanisms we have been talking about in my application to treating them. "What are you doing, balancing my membranes?" is the question. My answer, ?????.

Many of the things that I have observed working with you have assumed their rightful position, that of manifestations following a moment in space with the Breath of Life. The significance of where this spark chooses to demonstrate itself, according to individual need and potency, is truly amazing to watch and there is much to learn from it. If left to the Breath of Life, it may be only a whisper this time and occur within minutes after the beginning of observation, or it may be a spark that lights the room and occurs rapidly as it did for the woman with the miscarriage. Whatever the response, it is well to leave well enough alone. The Breath of Life knows its mechanisms–I am only the observer.

I would still like to know why I am having so much trouble with that one woman on whom I think I am missing the boat. Two questions: Can the Breath of Life be estranged from the body? What is the relation between withering fields and the Breath of Life? It is difficult to see why a small physical problem, such as a relatively fixed sacrum, would interfere so vitally with the full manifestation of the Breath of Life when the Breath of Life releases the problem so easily when it is ready to do so, and even until it is ready to do so, it prepares the tissues so it can release the mechanical fault. What is the relation between this mechanical fault and the Potent Breath of Life?

The things I am writing about I have observed, and I have done so without fanfare or verbal preparation of the patient, and the result for continued health is far more successful than with any other approach in the healing arts. Just ask my patients. I don't discuss this with them; they are satisfied to know that they are healing.

P.S. A thought strikes me: Could we call life a vital mechanical, mental, and emotional body operating ideally in a Still Breath of Life? With environmental stress within any phase, or combination of phases, there is formed a fulcrum of light providing the potency whereby that fulcrum maintains its pattern. The Light is neutral as to the reasons for and whereby such stresses are produced or maintained, but the Light is the fulcrum, and the force manifesting from it is the force that maintains the patterns. This applies emotionally, mentally and physically because when *any* change is made in the fulcrum, all three change their manifestations. In the correction of the fulcrum through that Light that centers it, the totality of body unity, in a Still Breath of Life as a unit in normal health, is again manifest.

Local areas of stress are merely maintained until the opportunity to return to the common pool of a common Breath of Life is again available.

The ideal is a Still Sea of Light. The less than ideal is wavelets or highlights in temporary manifestations of patterns as distinguished from the Still SeaAroundUs.

June 30, 1954

A thought struck me the other day while treating a patient, and it is a comment on a comment you made to some of us in Chicago at the time we went to see the show, *South Pacific*. The curtain partially occluded one of the scenes of the play, and your comment was that you wished the curtain would completely drop over the whole scene of action. The comment had to do with the fact that in the cranial mechanism, if the curtain (the curtain that I refer to in my dealings with you that has fallen across so many of my pet theories) would fall across the total mechanism, we would cease to be impressed with the machinery and see the reality. That comment came back to me the other day with the new interpretation and realization that in operating as close to the fulcrum as I can get, I certainly get a wonderful view of both ends of the lever, and the curtain is certainly closed and I can't see through it. Yet I still get a view through it that cannot be described. We thank you.

I also have a comment or two to make on explaining the so-called tissue reactions that take place in connective tissues for weeks after a treatment to "secure balance in these laws not framed by human hand." At one time I made the statement that a pattern of stress had to go back through its pattern of disability to recover, and this bright bit of information was rammed back into my throat. It was wrong. But here is a new version to explain some of this syndrome of healing. Here in Texas, we dumb cotton farmers plant cotton until we get no crop because we don't rebuild the soil. So we are told to plant vetch during the winter to rebuild the soil. We do it. The next spring we replant cotton, and the crop is a failure. The vetch is given the credit for the failure. We don't plant vetch the next winter, and the following spring we plant cotton again. We get a whale of a crop. Our conclusions: Plant vetch, no cotton crop; don't plant vetch, good cotton crop. Department of Agriculture conclusions: Plant vetch and the soil is so poor it takes all the following year to absorb the energy of the vetch and transform the nitrogen into the soil, and the next spring that nitrogen is available for use to grow cotton.

In cases of withering fields, could we use the same analogy?[16] As the waters of the brain are restored to living fascias that have been drought stricken, the first crops of functioning within the fascias express symptoms of revival towards normal water release and use, but

---

16. The term "withering fields" refers to Dr. Still's statement: "A thought strikes him that the cerebro spinal fluid is the highest known element that is contained in the human body, and unless the brain furnishes this fluid in abundance, a disabled condition of the body will remain. He who is able to reason will see that this great river of life must be tapped and the withering field irrigated at once, or the harvest of health be forever lost" (A.T. Still, *Philosophy of Osteopathy*, p. 39).

they haven't had water for a long time, and the first effect of this is expressed as symptoms.

The note on my card which I wrote to remind me to write you of this idea states: "Withering fields instilled with water make changes like renewing burned out cotton land with vetch." I think you have the idea I have in mind. I have two patients who have been thoroughly burned out withering fields for many years. They are now experiencing broad symptom complexes, and yet to my examination, I would say the Breath of Life is fully operating within an interchanging mechanism, and there are tremendous renewing changes occurring throughout their entire bodies.

A comment on my latest guess would be appreciated.

July 4, 1954   *Response from Dr. Sutherland*

Re: desired comment. Cleverly and intelligently stated. A true bale of cotton.

August 9, 1954

We have had a busy summer, and it continues to look as though it will not provide time to do the things that we want done—such as get all the weeds out of the lawn, try to keep cool, pay all the bills, and try to understand the fulcrum.

A comment on the Fulcrum: The sense world and its patterns do not react to the Fulcrum. A shift in the Fulcrum (and I mean Fulcrum with a capital "F") creates a new pattern. It isn't a mere change in the old one—the old one has gone. A new pattern is manifest in the sense and pattern world. The reason all this came to be commented upon is that one of our cranial colleagues has been ill for some time, and I have treated him daily. Being one of us, it is his idea that I should follow his patterns to get results, but when I do this, nothing permanent to benefit him occurs. I note that when the Fulcrum shifts, a correction has taken place. He continues to follow the pattern changes and attributes the improvement to them. I note a change in the Fulcrum is followed by new patterns. His health is returning. Needless to say, one of us is confused—I think it is me.

...A new D.O. was in the other day for a good long talk about the work we are doing. He had observed and watched me some, and we had an evening of explanation to try to clarify the picture. He was interested in trying to see what was the reason for some of my results, but...and "but" was as far as we could get together. He thought the answers ought to be clearly outlined, easy to read, with instructions for putting together available in six languages. How to make them see between the lines? I tried every trick I knew but:

Miracles not performed. Cures not guaranteed.

Professional skill to the best of our ability

the only guarantee!

September 12, 1954

Dr. Becker traveled to California in late August of 1954 to treat Dr. Sutherland, who was ailing at the time. This was his last visit with Dr. Sutherland before he died in November, 1954. For a description of one of Dr. Becker's experiences during that visit, see p. 240.

...The biggest thrill of the whole trip to me was the privilege of visiting and working with you folks in the Light that was present in your home and in the hospital. With the Potency that is present in that atmosphere and in your company, only the finest results can be obtained. The experience verifies the fact that working in the Knowing is a reality and as practical as drinking a glass of water. It is an experience that will never be forgotten. I am very grateful for the opportunity to have shared in it.

The following is a letter written to Dr. Becker by his mother.

November 26, 1954

Dear Rollin,

I drove to the post office to mail some letters and found your airmail note about Will Sutherland's passing. My first thought was how wonderful that he had you with him so near the last. I know it meant a lot to him, and now the bond between [the two of] you can still be of help to you. You have the spiritual insight to receive, and, as you receive, you will pass it on in physical demonstration.

You ask, "Why?" I can't answer, but I have the advantage that age brings and can see more plainly now than I could when I was young. I can accept whatever measure of good or insight there is in each person I come in contact with, knowing that each and every one of us is on the Divine Path somewhere, and those who seem blind to the truths which are clear to me just haven't been as fortunate as I. There must be a lot more advanced souls who view my struggles as those of a kindergarten student, but the more one advances, the more tolerant they become, so I don't mind.

I know what you mean exactly—the old story of being "scientific" about a spiritual truth. I wish I knew another word besides "spiritual"—its connotation limits it. The Indwelling Spirit—the Word—or as you say, The Breath of Life—well, dear, there are those you *can't* explain it to—you can't find a point of contact—so all you can do is to live it and let the Indwelling Presence guide your work. I know you do that, and of you people say, "I don't know what he's got, but it's something." Just so the patients get the benefit—that is all that counts. Once in a while somebody will understand....

Mother

14. CORRESPONDENCE: ANNE L. WALES, D.O.

These are edited excerpts from letters written by Dr. Becker to Anne L. Wales, D.O. Dr. Becker and Dr. Wales were both a part of Dr. Sutherland's associate faculty, and they served together over many years as members of the board of trustees of the Sutherland Cranial Teaching Foundation. Throughout that time, each considered the other to be a close colleague with whom they could share all of their thoughts.

March 8, 1956

Your paper is a beautiful description of the cranial concept, it is orderly, concise, and understandable (provided the reader has chosen a wide enough base with which to view the picture). You will note that I have penciled in a few minor ideas. One thing is I feel you need a more comprehensive term than "skeletal system" to indicate the depth of Will's view of the mechanism. You used the words "living biological organism" on the first page, and you could substitute these or similar words for skeletal system. You undoubtedly can find better ones.

I read an interesting editorial the other day on the subject of learning and it made sense to me in trying to say why we struggle so in getting Will's message across. The editorial pointed out that the learning process includes at least three factors: the ability to learn, the desire to learn, and material for learning. Will has given us a message that goes beyond or behind the curtain of the great mass of orthodox teaching processes. There are individuals who have the capacity for learning in his field of endeavor, but there is an even greater group who have not been introduced to the idea that such type of learning is even possible. This group has to awaken to such a process first, then they must create a desire to learn about such things within themselves, and then they are ready for the material that is available for them.... It sure is a slow climb to reach a point to where we can say, now let us begin to study the message of Dr. Will Sutherland. Beginnings, always beginnings. When do we ever reach a point when we can say we have arrived? I can see why they call the giving of college degrees commencement exercises. It seems to me I am forever commencing.

I am increasingly conscious of the tremendous work there is to be done to make "these laws not framed by human hand" understood.[1] We are going to have to develop a whole new terminology in words that describe function instead of end products. Present-day laws describe the final products, not the processes that produced them, and Will's laws deal with the processes that produce end products. What a field for research! Where does one start? How does one keep the whole picture in mind as one adds one factor after another? How does one continually integrate as he picks up more pieces to fill out the picture? How does one learn to avoid blind alleys, or rather how does one keep to the main avenue and make adequate examination of all the streets that lead into it? Quite a job.

April 5, 1967

...There is a tremendous difference between talking about the Breath of Life in the Science of Osteopathy and putting it to work on a consistent basis in *every* patient with *every* treatment....

...I well recall when I was studying under Will and I would bring a problem to him to which he would respond, "Why not?" It took me five years to learn his "Why not?" meant, "Rollin, you are out in left field. Start all over." When I would finally iron out an answer that did fulfill the need, he made no reply at all; he would merely smile at me. If I had the answer and he knew the answer, what was there to discuss?

---

1. "I do not claim to be the author of this science of Osteopathy. No human hand framed its law; I ask no greater honor than to have discovered it" (A.T. Still, *Autobiography*, p. 302).

April 2, 1969

I had an experience last Friday night at the Academy [of Applied Osteopathy] talk that I want to pass on to you. There were 78 doctors signed up for the three-day meeting, and Friday evening, the meeting was split into two groups, one to hear Dr. Angus Cathie on "Frozen Shoulders" and the other to hear Becker on "Still's Principles of Palpation." About 25 listened to my talk and 12 of them stayed to practice the work given them afterwards.

As you know, I started talking about "diagnostic touch," "biokinetic energies," "biodynamic energies," and "potency" about eight years ago, and you are the only one who ever commented that they liked the terminology or the descriptive analysis. So Friday night, I left out all those terms in my talk.[2]

I explained to them that for 8 years I had used the manipulative osteopathy taught to me in school and post-graduate work and that I became disenchanted with my use of it because I could not control or know why cases did or did not make the type of recovery I expected. Driven by this disenchantment, I went back to Dr. Still's *Autobiography* and relearned his basic principles. Two years later, in 1944, I studied under Dr. Sutherland and learned the detailed anatomy and physiology of the craniosacral mechanism, which completed my knowledge of the total body physiology. I gradually developed the type of diagnostic and therapeutic approach I use today. I told them that I had given this type of care in more than 60,000 treatment programs and that I have used it in practically every type of clinical problem a busy physician sees in his practice—every kind of trauma, disease, and clinical entity.

I then gave them two quotations from Dr. Still's *Autobiography*:

I hope all who may read after my pen will see that I am fully convinced that God, of the mind of nature, has proven His ability to plan

---

2. Dr. Becker wrote a series of articles entitled, "Diagnostic Touch: Its Principles and Application." These papers were originally published in the 1963–65 *Yearbooks* of the Academy of Applied Osteopathy (currently called the American Academy of Osteopathy). They appear in an edited form in Dr. Becker's *Life in Motion*.

(if plan be necessary) and to make or furnish laws of self, without patterns, for the myriads of forms of animated beings; and to thoroughly equip them for the duties of life, with their engines and batteries of motor force all in action. Each part is fully armed for duty, empowered to select and appropriate to itself from the great laboratory of nature such forces as are needed to enable it to discharge the duties peculiar to its office in the economy of life. [pp. 148–49]

For about twelve months I have been busily engaged in overhauling my loom. I have a loom of the finest construction; not made on Earth, neither is it made by hand.... By the ability they [the threads] contain, it is only necessary for me to start the loom in motion. [pp. 318–19]

The first quotation indicated that the motor forces were already in action in living anatomy, and the second quote said that all I had to do was start the loom in motion and the pattern of disability would be laid out for my palpatory observation.

Finally, I gave them the instruction that they had to be *active* in their palpatory examination and work with the living anatomy and with the physiological changes taking place under their hands. Those that stayed for the practice session all felt living anatomy at work and the corrections that took place. These corrections, by the way, take place usually within ten minutes during any treatment program.

With this brief summary, my point is this: Physicians in the field do not like to have new terminology thrown at them. They want clear explanations in the language which they are using in their everyday practice. I do not plan to use the term "diagnostic touch" in future discussions of Still's and Sutherland's basic principles of anatomy and physiology and the palpatory skills it takes to bring these into clinical use.

The material I sent you is valid, however. It is simple to use after you acquire a *knowing* sense of touch, and it gives you practically 100% control for each clinical problem during each visit made by the patient. It will keep you informed as to the therapeutic progress, gain or loss, and it will permit the greatest reversibility of pathology possible for any given condition. Even if you, as a trained physician with modern-day understanding, don't think reversibility is possible, this approach may prove itself to be helpful in spite of what you think. Irreversible problems will not resolve themselves, and you will be given insight into these matters so that you will know why they do not respond.

I have been invited to talk in Kirksville on the same subject, and I have asked them to call the talk "Osteopathic Palpation" instead of "Diagnostic Touch." I call this terminology issue to your attention because you are interested in writing for others.

...I was interested in your description of the treatment *you* received when you treated your patient. I am convinced that when we tap into the potency within our patients and go *through* it during the treatment program, we, too, receive a treatment. Since the normal for the patient and the normal for ourselves *always* wants to manifest itself, we get benefit from using this approach whether we are conscious of it or not.

...Yes, "*consent* to be *used*" is a most useful thought. There are not too many who will appreciate it. I know you do appreciate this thought of mine, but I have run into road blocks when I try it out on others. This, too, is something I plan to use cautiously in future presentations.

August 26, 1970

I may not have learned as much as I should have in regards to learning terminology that works in talking to others who do the work we do, but I certainly have been taught much for my own use in my conceptual thinking and action. [The journal] *Main Currents in Modern Thought* is valuable to me.[3]

---

3. Published from 1940–75. Originally published by the Center for Integrated Education, New Rochelle, New York., it was later published by Gordon & Breach.

January 23, 1974

It is interesting to me that in the total functioning of the body, there are, basically, two types of motility and mobility—voluntary and involuntary. The voluntary is that which we project through our sensory and motor systems—there is input and output. The involuntary is even more remarkable in that it is strictly a matter of flexion and extension for midline structures and external and internal rotation for bilateral structures for everything from the fluids to the bony skeleton. Each and every individual portion of the body is designed and coordinated by its individual shape and contours to manifest flexion/external rotation and extension/internal rotation. Therefore it is necessary to study the interrelationship of the fluids, soft tissues, and bony contours in their involuntary movements. All the involuntary mechanisms are moving in the same, simple, primary way throughout the body, whether it be at rest or in voluntary motion. If I can restore the involuntary mobility and motility, bringing it to its full potential in my treatment of my patient, the voluntary mechanisms will automatically correct themselves.

February 19, 1974

You are welcome to use the paragraph concerning voluntary and involuntary mobility and motility of the human body. As a clinical entity to literally be used in diagnosis and treatment, it is practically an unknown factor among the profession. The "cranial" group has learned about it in regard to the primary respiratory mechanism, but they usually stop there. If they use it at all, they do not consider it for the total body physiology in their thinking or their actions.

June 2, 1976

You got me to thinking...about our colleagues in the cranial field who do not understand this "foreign language." I think it has always been hard to accept the fact that the "fluid drive," sparked into action by a Breath of Life, is the true fundamental principle of the primary respiratory mechanism. The fluid drive, the motile central nervous system, the Sutherland fulcrum and reciprocal tension membrane, and the cranial bones and sacrum that go along for the ride are all dependent on this "Spark" and the resultant fluid drive. I don't blame our colleagues. It's a tough nut to chew on, although it is simple, as Will said.

...P.S. All of us, including all of our colleagues, have been using these principles in our treatment programs, because that is the only way in which it can work. The acceptance of *why* it works this way has been much harder to envision.

January 27, 1979

The assignment given to me for the SCTF [Sutherland Cranial Teaching Foundation] Conference is, "Motion—The Key to Diagnosis and Treatment."[4] It seems to be a simple enough title to talk about, but where does one start when so much has already been said about it? I had a thought the other day that I would like to share with you. Several years ago I became aware of an additional tide-like movement of the total body physiology in addition to the rhythmic ten-to-fourteen-times-a-minute movement of the craniosacral rhythm. It is a much slower, total rhythm of the total body physiology, which takes place about six times in a ten-minute period of time. It is a more massive-feeling Tide with a gradual welling expansion of the whole being and a gradual receding movement, which is followed by another gradual, massive expansion in rhythmic interchange within and throughout the total organism.

It is a powerful therapeutic tool, and like the cerebrospinal fluid fluctuation, it can be used with so-called "Tide control." When I, the physician, can share this slow, majestic rhythm subjectively with the patient during the treatment, from within-out, there is a total interchange throughout the physiology of the patient. Interchanging with what? I have no idea as to the source of this slow rhythm nor of its basic nature. I do know that when I take the time to let this slow

---

4. This paper appears in an edited form in Dr. Becker's *Life in Motion*.

rhythm do its work within the patient, it accomplishes more towards physiological rebalancing than anything I have ever observed in any other form of treatment. It is not separate from and cannot be considered independent from all the other patterns of the body—all the other voluntary and involuntary mechanisms. It is part and parcel of the total function within each of us.

Palpation: The art of palpation can be viewed as including palpation for the voluntary functioning of the body physiology from without-in and palpation for the involuntary functioning of body physiology from within-out. Additionally, I feel there is an even deeper art of palpation than the voluntary or involuntary. That deeper art is a subjective form of palpation in which the subjective awareness of the physician fuses with the patient's subjective awareness of his/her total body physiology and thereby shares the experience of the patient's total involuntary functioning. It is this latter experience that allows this slow rhythm to demonstrate its working within the patient and to coordinate its work through a treatment session.

April 27, 1981

This must be a blue Monday. I have had a tough time trying to keep from shooting the patients instead of treating them. "This, too, shall pass," I hope.

January 23, 1987

While reading your manuscript[5], I had a feeling of reliving a period of my life from 1944 to 1954 in which I shared time with you, Chester, Will, and Adah.[6] There were many Highs and Lows and through them all were the steadfastness and the Guiding Light of WGS along with his knowledge of the primary respiratory mechanism of a living Science of Osteopathy. Now comes another generation of doctors who

----

5. W.G. Sutherland, *Teachings in the Science of Osteopathy*, edited by Anne L. Wales.
6. Chester Handy, D.O. (1911–1963) was Dr. Wales' husband and a member of Dr. Sutherland's associate faculty. "Will" and "Adah" refers to Dr. and Mrs. Sutherland.

need to keep that growth alive through our and the SCTF's dedication to Will's basic teaching.[7] Some of our younger generation want to write their own ticket instead of *listening*. I am glad we have an Anne Wales who is *Listening* and getting the message reactivated.

...Will wanted his work to be a true study of the primary respiratory mechanism within a True Science of Osteopathy. He had it, he studied it, he experienced it, he knew it. He wanted each individual to *live* it with him.

August 21, 1987

...You made a statement to the effect that when Will showed up in New York, you chose to follow Will and devote your life to make his work live. You have spent as many years to do his work as it took Will to try to get it out to the profession.

Will took from 1900 to 1944—you have taken from 1944 to 1987. It was worth the trip and we are grateful that your one-on-one relationship with Will was a story of love and devotion....

---

7. Dr. Becker was president of the Sutherland Cranial Teaching Foundation (SCTF) from 1962 to 1979 and served on its board of trustees from the 1950's to 1988.

15. Correspondence: Colleagues and Friends

These are edited excerpts from letters written by Dr. Becker to various colleagues and friends.

October 27, 1955

Dear Adah [Mrs. Sutherland],

...Regardless of how you spell it or try to explain it, the Fulcrum and its centering Boss is still the only approach to health and disease. With increasing awareness of its potency, I am more impressed every day in patient after patient, problem after problem. If one is aware of it, one doesn't need to exclaim over it and if one can't seem to be aware of it, you just can't explain it.

I was very interested in a new book, *The Unified System Concept of Nature* by Stephen Bornemisza [1955], in which he evaluates all of nature—inanimate and animate objects—into a common pattern of expression. It is an interesting analysis of what is happening, and were he to say each and every change he analyzes is centered by fulcrums, he would add the final touch. As one reads his work with that thought in mind, it certainly shows the similarity between physics and biology.

Another factor that keeps cropping into my awareness is the necessity to cover the material aspect with a curtain. So much more goes on behind that curtain than can be appreciated until the curtain rolls back and reveals the new relationships that have been developed.[1]

I am convinced that we need to take Will's life work, translate it into present-day terminology and get it into the heads of our present-day students. It loses none of its potency and would be infinitely

---

1. For an explanation of the phrase, "behind the curtain," see p. 240.

more palatable. However, the big problem is that with awareness of his message, there is no terminology that is adequate to explain it. The words of his day were inadequate and today's are equally so. But at least we could describe the mechanics of his findings in present-day physical and biological terms, as did Bornemisza, and let the physician studying these terms realize the potential of the centering fulcrum. Another difficulty is that most of us have no idea that we are to turn another page. We are too satisfied with our present concepts....

December 21, 1955
Dear Adah,

...I am also supposed to discuss technique, but how can I when I have none except the living body on which I am working?

November 2, 1961
Dear Dr. ——,

Your very interesting letter and manuscript ask for comments but I am at a quandary as to how to comment. I have drawn a sketch that George Laughlin handed to me the last night I was in Kirksville. He asked, "Isn't there a basic potency within everyone that represents the total health of the individual?" My answer was, "Yes. In fact when you study the individual under your hands and read through to his basic potency, you will discover that it wants to go into action and both the disease potencies and the traumatic potencies tend to dissipate, leaving only the basic potency to carry on the job of maintaining health." He nodded his head and that was the end of the discussion.

There is this basic potency that is as perceptible to the understanding touch as is the potency of an injury or of a disease. The disease and traumatic potencies are easier to find because they function in a more or less definite focus depending on the patient's disabilities.

But the basic potency is there and is the dominant one in every sense of the word. It can be perceived and initiated into action with every diagnostic and therapeutic effort.

Your "vital force body" and its relationship to the "dense physical organism" is an apt description which could very easily be true. I wouldn't know. In this work, as you and I are trying to develop our understanding, each individual works up an idea to express that which we are trying to understand. For you, what you have described may be an excellent approach. Someone else may find an analogy which suits them better. I do know this, there is a basic power within each one of us that is doing its best to keep us healthy and in tune with the universe around us. It can be perceived by knowing hands and knowing minds. It can be used to bring back health. We should try to create understanding within ourselves of this great power and at the same time not let our limited verbalizations of our understanding limit our experience in using this power by trying to make it fit our conception of it. This basic power is a lot bigger and smarter than we are and I am for letting it take the lead in developing my understanding of it.

I am not in any sense of the word criticizing your comments. I like them. They show understanding and insight. They show knowledge of more to be learned. They show knowledge that you know there is more to be learned. All I know is that you are cooking in the right kitchen. When you get some more details, I sure would like to have them.

At my recent talk in Kirksville, I did not mention the basic potency and the ability of the physician to find it because it is so much easier to find the disease and traumatic potencies. After one has spent time finding these lesser lights, all of a sudden one day, he is conscious that there is a much brighter light within his patient that far outshines the ones associated with disease or trauma. It has been there all the time, but it takes time to know it. So I confined my talk to that which could be more easily perceived. If any of us ever gets our start into this field, we are led to the basic potency. But we have to start somewhere.

Where the C.R.I. [cranial rhythmic impulse] comes into the picture does create a dilemma. It is another reading like the blood pressure or blood count. I am in total agreement with your statement: "...but the observations described herein extend above and beyond this C.R.I."

Editor's note: The statement in the physician's letter is as follows. "...Comparison between the vital forces described and the cranial rhythmic impulse is difficult to delineate. The cranial rhythmic impulse is undoubtedly the physical manifestation of the vital forces at work, but the observations described herein extend above and beyond this C.R.I."

Mid-1960's

Dear Dr.——,

I have a thought that came through to me about two weeks ago, which I think is worth your consideration. The fact that it took 34 years of clinical experience in order to be able to deliver the thought does not necessarily mean that all gestation periods have to be that long. The thought is basically this: There are postural patterns or dynamics of functioning within each individual that are individualized for that particular person and for no other person on Earth.

Just as there are homeostatic controls over the general systems of the body that only permit physiological functioning within certain limits, and just as we have immune reactions to all foreign cells that enter our bodies, so it is that there is a postural entity, a dynamic postural pattern that is specific for each individual. This is a dynamic pattern of functioning.

This postural pattern begins prenatally in the formation of the body within the physical environment of the uterus. The pattern is further modified by the birth processes. It continues to be developed through the growing years from babyhood to childhood to adulthood. It involves every cell of the musculoskeletal system and every cell of the total connective tissue framework of the body, training itself to become the postural entity in structure and function that is correct for that one individual.

In the case of the body's general systems and its immune reaction to foreign substances, any deviation from normal physiological functioning causes the body to immediately react to restore homeostasis by hormonal and chemical means. Likewise in response to any event that takes the body out of its normal postural pattern of functioning, the body immediately makes efforts to correct this problem. It works to restore the normal pattern of functioning that has been built into the connective tissue framework, the enclosed musculature and ligaments, and the osseous skeleton around which this mechanism is formed.

To carry this into the clinical field, if you were to see a group of patients with a fifth lumbar strain who all apparently have the same type of strain, you would discover you will never see a strain identical with the one that is in the patient that comes to you for diagnosis and treatment. In each case, this is a strain pattern that has broken the rules. It has broken away from the postural pattern of this particular patient and is seeking aid to restore it to the normal pattern factor of function that is right for that one individual.

The dynamics of the postural pattern within every individual are such that they are constantly seeking to restore, from the top of the head to the soles of the feet, the pattern around which that person has existed from before birth. We as osteopathic physicians are trying to assist that body to return something to normal. It already knows it is normal and merely requires our assistance to effect the changes the body is seeking. A gross manipulation of this particular area is a generalized help for the particular problem. But a more specific treatment requires the specific analysis of: What is the postural pattern that is right for this one individual? Treatment is then applied toward the restoration of this functioning pattern. The aim is to aid the body in this particular area to adapt itself back to its normal pattern.

This is not a new thought necessarily. It is, perhaps, a restatement of an old thought we have known for years. I believe it could be *one* of the tangibles that you are seeking in the search for a new tangible. I would appreciate your comments.

June 3, 1974

Dear —,

...I then decided to start all over again. Thus, I reread Andrew Taylor Still's original writings, especially his *Autobiography* and his *Philosophy of Osteopathy*. Furthermore, in 1944, I began learning cranial osteopathy under the direction of William Sutherland. And so gradually I gathered the methods that I use today by borrowing Still's and Sutherland's principles and reincorporating them into the human body's entire anatomical-physiological structure.

...In terms of attempting to explain my therapeutic approach to patients, I do not even try. As I was perfecting my diagnostic and treatment methods as well as my comprehension of the pathological states presented to me, I realized that my patients did not try to understand how I worked; what interested them was to have results that alleviated and resolved their problems. By placing my hands and my Silent Partner in contact with the areas of complaint, I delved into the reason for their difficulties. This way, instead of explaining to them "how" I worked, I was able to explain the "why" of their problems. And this satisfied them.

...A study of the enclosed documents will help you to understand and experiment with what we will do when you come to Dallas next January. It is a method that will demand an ever continuing-faith. Take your time with it and keep it simple. You have the rest of your life to master it.

October 28, 1976

Dear Dr. —,

Thank you for sending me a copy of your paper.... I agree with it in principle in that it is necessary to take the energy field into action along with the physical parts involved in somatic dysfunction. But both the energy field and the tissue involvement are merely effects and not causes....

In the latter part of the paper you speak about manipulating this energy field. If I were to experience the same treatment results you described, I would have to ask myself, "Did I *manipulate* this energy field or did I *observe* this energy field making changes?" Let me illustrate: A twisted fishing line with a light weight on it or a twisted telephone cord are twisted and have distorted energy fields associated with them. I hold up the fishing line or telephone cord, and the lines unwind themselves and correct the line and distortion fields. Did I manipulate them or observe them?

February 17, 1978
Dear Faculty Member:

...I would like to make a few comments on the osseous elements of the skull. The osseous elements are *living* plates of bone, intimately in contact with the RTM [reciprocal tension membrane], which are complex in their shape, in their interdigitations with each other, and in their mobility patterns. Like multiple cogged wheels, move any one of them in the neurocranium or face, and every *living* bone in the whole complex has to accommodate the change of position and function of the moved bone. In addition the RTM patterns in turn are modified by the changes in these living bones, and the fluid drive of the CSF and the CNS are modified. This applies to the everyday accommodations to walking, moving about, leaning our chin on our hand, etc. The movements and compressions of the osseous elements cannot be separated from the RTM that lines them, and the rhythmic movements of the RTM directly involve every minor and major movement of the osseous elements. Detailed *knowledge* of *all* elements of the total involuntary mechanisms share in importance in our understanding of anatomy and physiology.

May 16, 1978
Dear Swami Ram Baba,

First, I want to express what a pleasure and a privilege it was to meet you and to share the short time we were together at Dan's place and in our home. I felt an instant rapport, a "rhythmic balanced interchange," with you, as did my wife, Ardath, and the feeling continues.

For you, this may be a common experience, but it is an uncommon experience in the years I have been meeting individuals. Yes, there have been a limited few, so, maybe, that is the reason I recognized the one we shared with you.

...I have acquired two more cancer cases in my practice since you left. I would like to describe my approach in these cases and ask if you can suggest anything else I could add to their care. I am *not* the primary physician in any of these cases. They have other physicians for their diagnosis, their operations, their medicines, their chemotherapy, etc. They come to me for supplemental care. I do not even ask them the nature of the cancer.

I treat them as follows: I AM an Empty Bowl in the presence of my Maker, I know the patient to be an Empty Bowl in the same Presence, I place my hands under various areas of stress (much as I did with you) and work until "I" get orders that the treatment is through for that day. Most of these people come to me about once a week or every two weeks as I feel that it takes time for each treatment to do its work for the patients. That is it. Any suggestions?

Dan was kind enough to give me a skull cup from a Lama [who had lived] about 150 to 200 years ago. It is most unusual in that the meditations he had performed had thinned the vertex of his skull to a singular layer of bone instead of the usual two layers. Truly, matter and energy are interchangeable....

July 22, 1978

Dear Dr. ——,

...Yes, your whole practice life, and probably your life itself, has a new road to follow–and it is great.

Allow me to give you a quote from W. G. Sutherland: "Allow physiological function within to manifest its own unerring potency rather than using blind force from without....A potency that has within it an Intelligence, spelled with a capital I...."

When I began to work with the inner resources of the patient through the application of the basic principles given to us by Drs.

Still and Sutherland, I ran into the same problem of patients with overloads or underloads who either zapped me or drained me. I asked Dr. Sutherland about it and he said, "That is true and it is not necessary. You have the right to protect yourself." He did not tell me how.

Through the years I learned that I have a Silent Partner, a Source, and my patient has a Silent Partner, his or her Source—a Source that supplies all the potency needed for my walk about on Earth, the same one that my patient has within him or her.

Therefore, I tune into my Silent Partner, first, and, silently through my Silent Partner, I tune into the Silent Partner of the patient and suggest to the Silent Partner of the patient that they use their own Source for their potency needs.

I am no longer taking a roller coaster ride of getting zaps from overloads or giving to underloads. My Source and their Source are the same Source and each of us are protected and meeting our specific needs.

May your new road give you peace and pleasure.

July 20, 1981

Dear ——,

My sincere thanks for the chapter from Joel S. Goldsmith's work. I especially like his book *The Mystical I.*

Last June at the SCTF [Sutherland Cranial Teaching Foundation] Conference, I gave a talk with the following statement as the topic for discussion, "The unity of function includes power, matter, motion and time as a continuum." The definition of "continuum" is: "A continuous whole, quantity, or series; a thing whose parts cannot be separately discerned."

The word, "power," referred to the same word as defined and used by Joel Goldsmith, although I did not mention his name to the group. Matter, motion, and time are obviously the manifesting elements of the unity of function as a continuum.

I like the writings of Joel Goldsmith because there is no middle man. It is strictly a one-with-one relationship between me and my Maker.

October 22, 1982

Dear——,

...You ask for suggestions as to how to study the cranial mechanism in more detail. Get a disarticulated skull and make it a good-quality bony skull. Learn to rearticulate it as a unit and continue to refine your knowledge of how each piece and articulation moves in flexion and/or external rotation and extension and/or internal rotation, depending on whether it is midline or bilateral. Know and feel at all times that the neurocranial bones are on *one* reciprocal tension membrane that moves the cranial bones (all of them) and controls the range of movement of each of them. Picture this on the disarticulated skeleton and in the living head.

That is a start for getting a picture of the whole mechanism in reciprocal movement. Then one can go to local areas, looking at what is happening to a temporal bone in a patient you see that has problems in that area, and so it goes deeper and deeper.

I spent a lot of time in my early years with my disarticulated skull. Ask [my wife] Ardath.

April 1, 1986

Dear Dr. ——,

I am glad you are taking such an interest in the science of osteopathy....I am enclosing some of the basic material that allows me to "understand the mechanism" in preparation for a "technique" for treatment purposes. First is the basic definition of the science of osteopathy in one paragraph, which I read in Still's autobiography and which I accepted, without question.[2] I accepted Still's description of a living mechanism available for my *use* in diagnosis and treatment. I had practiced general OMT [osteopathic manipulative treatment] for ten years, found it wanting in understanding and clinical results. Then I found that paragraph, gave up my general OMT and used the material in that definition to develop my knowledge and use of the *livingness*

---

2. For the full quotation see p. 3.

of the body physiology and the patient's own self-correction towards health from within.

The key is to accept what is in that paragraph without question, to develop an inner degree of palpatory skill with which to read the body physiology of the patient, and to "allow physiological function within (the patient) to manifest its own unerring potency, rather than the use of blind force from without." (W.G. Sutherland)

...I have been using this approach for the past 42 years and am still learning. As soon as the patient enters my office, I become a student, the "physician-within" the patient becomes the teacher, and his/her body physiology becomes the living tools through which my palpatory skills can learn to "understand the mechanism" for that given day. As soon as my hands and body contacts have been made, I begin to feel, to listen, to quietly, without judgment, actively experience what the physician within and the body physiology of the patient is manifesting through my palpatory contacts. When this diagnostic-treatment session is finished, I can remove my palpatory contacts and then "think" about what took place. To analyze with judgment during the treatment session inhibits some of the material the living moving body physiology is trying to give to you.

To actively, quietly "listen" through your palpatory contacts is to receive many interesting experiences. To position your palpatory contacts and then think about everything else, or not try to listen to the "teacher" within the patient, is to experience nothing during the time you should be "listening." Prove this to yourself—make your palpatory contacts and actively "listen," without judgment, and then quit listening and note the difference in what you are experiencing from within the body physiology of the patient. To actively "listen" is to gain experience in learning to "know the mechanism," and each patient is an excellent teacher. To not "listen" provides no living contacts and no information for the body physiology to give to you. Turn on your quiet listening and stay with it through the whole diagnostic-treatment time.

Enough for now. The next patient is opening your door for you to experience their problem and/or health mechanism. Go to work.

16. Stories of Dr. Becker

These are stories that were related to this editor. The first two were told by Dr. Becker; the third one, by John Harakal, D.O.

If You Understand the Mechanism

Towards the end of his life, Dr. Sutherland suffered from a very painful condition of his foot. Two months before Dr. Sutherland's death, Dr. Becker went to visit him hoping to render any help he could. Dr. Becker found that he was able to provide Dr. Sutherland with some hours of pain relief through the use of osteopathic manipulative treatment, and he did this over the course of several days.

Dr. Becker's plans called for him to depart for some days and then to return to see Dr. Sutherland again. Before leaving, Dr. Becker showed another colleague who had come to visit, what he had been doing to successfully relieve Dr. Sutherland's suffering.

Upon Dr. Becker's return, he found Dr. Sutherland moaning in pain, with the distraught colleague saying that he had done just what Dr. Becker had shown him to do, but to no avail. The doctor said he couldn't understand why it hadn't worked, at which point Dr. Sutherland stopped moaning, abruptly sat up, and exclaimed, "If you understand the mechanism, the technique is simple."

Behind the Curtain

In the correspondence between Dr. Becker and Dr. Sutherland, they often expressed the idea that something had "gone behind the curtain." Dr. Becker related the following story by way of explanation.

Dr. Becker had been struggling for some time with the understanding of a particular concept and had gotten to the point where he was

drawing some conclusions. With this in mind, he was eagerly antici-
pating an upcoming meeting with Dr. Sutherland at a conference they
would both be attending. There, Dr. Becker would have a chance to
discuss the issue with him in order to see if he had arrived at some
true understanding.

Arriving at the conference, Dr. Becker spent some hours with another one of his colleagues discussing and refining his thinking on
this idea. Finally, the time came for Dr. Becker to go to Dr. Sutherland's
hotel room. Once there, to Dr. Becker's great amazement and dis-
tress, he experienced his mind as a total blank. He could not bring
forth a single thought on the subject he had prepared so thoroughly
to discuss. He asked Dr. Sutherland, "What is happening? Where did
it go?"

Dr. Sutherland replied, "It has gone behind the curtain and is now
available for use."

⌐ ⌐ ⌐

Among Dr. Becker's writings is the following statement:

Teaching is an art and a science wherein the material presented
goes behind the curtain and allows the student to become a beholder,
developing his own understanding from within.

Where Was Your Attention?

Dr. Becker and Dr. Harakal were fishing one afternoon, as they
regularly did. They had been on a small private lake owned by a friend,
and at the end of the day, they had to hike up through a pasture to get
back to their car on the road. As they were packing up their gear
beside the lake, Dr. Harakal noticed there was a big bull standing in
the pasture.

Dr. Becker finished with his gear and strode up to the road. The
bull took no notice of Dr. Becker as he went by. A short time later,
Dr. Harakal started up through the pasture, keeping a watchful eye
on the bull. To his dismay, the bull started moving towards him in
what seemed a threatening way. Dr. Harakal quickened his pace and

thankfully made it to the road before the bull got too close.

When Dr. Harakal met up with Dr. Becker, he asked, "Why didn't the bull come after you? How come he went after me?"

Dr. Becker responded with the question, "Where was your attention?"

Dr. Harakal said, "On the bull. Where was yours?"

Pointing to himself, Dr. Becker answered, "Mine was inside."

17. SELF-TREATMENT APPROACHES

CHRONIC SINUSITIS
Dr. Becker sent this to a colleague in the 1980's.

A HOME TREATMENT FOR chronic sinusitis that is quite successful is as follows:

1) While sitting in a chair and facing a table, have the patient place his or her two first finger pads on the bridge of the nose, the nasal bones, so that the fingers contact each other and also contact the lower edge of the frontal bone at the metopic suture. The forefinger pads are basically on the nasal bones, not on the frontal processes of the maxillae.

2) Have the elbows rest on the table for stability.

3) Raise the shoulders and/or head cephalad (towards the ceiling) so as to *lightly* increase the pressure contacts of the forefingers on the nasal bones. Continue to hold this light pressure contact for a period of seven minutes. Have a clock in view so as to maintain this treatment cycle for the seven-minute period.

Physiology: The anterior superior pole of the reciprocal tension membrane (the falx cerebri's attachment to the crista galli) has been anchored so as to allow the fluctuation of the cerebrospinal fluid, the central nervous system motility, and the reciprocal tension membrane mobility to physiologically rock the mobility of all the "plumber's friends" to each sinus in the facial mechanisms for at least 70 cycles in a seven-minute period.

Editor's note: "Plumber's friend" is a colloquial term for the stick with a rubber cup on the end used to pump out clogged toilets. In Life in Motion *(p. 348), Dr. Becker writes: "There is a plumber's friend which literally pumps each of the sinuses.... For the maxillary sinus [it] is the zygomatic bone; for the sphenoidal sinus, it is the vomer." He describes the perpendicular plate of the ethmoid as the plumber's friend for the frontal sinus, with that same rocking motion acting on the ethmoid sinus.*

It has been my observation that there is marked improvement in chronic sinusitis cases if this approach is used at least once a day for 30 days. Continued daily, the healthy layers of mucosal sinus cells will come to the surface in about three months. The surface layer of mucosal cells in chronic sinusitis only know how to produce lots of mucus; the healthy mucosa takes time to deliver itself to the surface.

Keep it simple. It works.

I AM IN SILENCE

These are instructions that Dr. Becker gave to some of his patients for self-treatment. At times he gave this exercise on its own, at other times he gave it in conjunction with Robert Fulford, D.O.'s "book exercise."[1]

I AM IN SILENCE

Assume a position of comfort for a minimum period of ten minutes.

Allow the breath to come and go in rhythmic cycles without conscious effort.

Allow Consciousness or Awareness (without physical, emotional, or mental effort) to manifest

I AM SILENCE

for ten minutes.

Allow any physical, emotional, or mental effects that choose to come through to do so without effort and without placing the attention upon them. Let them be as clouds drifting across a clear sky. I AM SILENCE through the ten minutes without interruption as these effects pass through.

KEEP IT SIMPLE

---

1. See "Resting Spinal Stretch" in S.M. Davidson, *The Twig Unbent.*

What follows is a version of "I AM IN SILENCE" that was in Dr. Becker's personal papers. He credited the phrase to Walter Starcke (The Gospel of Relativity, 1973).

Be Still and Know that I AM God
or
I AM IN SILENCE

A ten-minute program to seek or try to experience Omnipotency, Omnipresence, and Omniscience:

Assume a posture or a position in which you can be in a state of comfort for a minimum period of ten minutes.

Allow the breathing to come in short rhythmic cycles of inhalation and exhalation without conscious effort.

Be Consciously Aware of seeking Stillness or Silence, not physically, *not* emotionally, *not* mentally, but with a deep inner Awareness of Consciously seeking Stillness or Silence for the total ten-minute period.

Allow any physical, emotional, or mental effects that choose to come through, to focus, or to pass through your being to do so without effort on your part and without any of your attention on their part. Let them be as clouds drifting across a clear sky. YOU maintain your Conscious Awareness of Stillness or Silence through the ten-minute period without interruption as these effects pass through you.

Use this program at least once a day or as often as you choose to do it in your daily schedule.

KEEP IT SIMPLE

18. REFLECTIONS AND INSIGHTS

These are excerpts from the notebooks in which Dr. Becker kept many of his written thoughts and ideas. Dates are included where he noted them. Dr. Becker freely incorporated the words of others into his private writings, which makes it difficult to draw a discrete line between his own words and those of the people who inspired him.

IF WE WANT TO understand this mechanism, we have to understand and feel how it functions in both a state of health and a state of illness. We have to learn *through it*; we must function as it functions; we must think as it thinks; and we have to experience it with our hands. We have to experience it in terms of its living function, understanding the way this body would act if it were in good health. We must not only explore symptoms; we have to look around, everywhere, across this living body, and find what *it* would like to be and how *it* would like to live. (1974)

The human body is in reciprocal balance with the whole universe and is individualized in the internal and external environmental response to the universe.

Therefore, one develops his touch to share with the biodynamic and biokinetic experience of the patients' bodies and their potencies—to become one with them in the moving stream of time, to guide them, to work with them, to follow through to the fulfillment that is available for *this time* and contact—to be them for the brief time they do their work, knowing they were already functioning when they were contacted and knowing they continue to function when released.

Let us assume that the physician and the patient are a "still" empty bowl as one unit. Let us assume the hands of the physician are a "still" empty bowl in contact with the patient allowing the contents of the patient to find "balance in those laws not framed by human hands."[1] Let the hands of the physician be a "nonresistance" sensomotor palpatory skill in contact with "Stillness" as the health patterns of the patient deliver themselves to anatomicophysiological function.

The tensity in the anatomicophysiological function of the patient requires sufficient palpatory skills by the physician to set up a "nonresistant" pattern to allow the tensity to dissipate to "Stillness," to go through "Stillness," to create movement in patterns towards health functioning (corrections usually take place between treatments, not at the time of treatment).

Traumatic energy is dissipated and/or disease energy is transmuted to maximum efficiency to go through the disease process to restore health.

A Healing Principle in Homeodynamics

Health is relatively free from inertia. Disease states or homeodynamic problems always involve inertia, for the problem itself is sustaining itself within its own energy field. A treatment program that utilizes the healing energies of the body has to overcome this inertia at treatment time before physical changes take place.

The age of the disease process affects the inertia. A chronic problem like hepatitis would be different than an acute process such as pneumonia.

The age of the patient is another major concern in dealing with the inertia of utilizing the living healing principles of the body. Age creates an inertia which must be waited through at treatment time before the fulcra display themselves. Compare the inertia of a 20- or 30-year-old with hepatitis and a 60-year-old with the same problem. It will take two to three times as long: 20 years—5 minutes; 60 years—12 to 15 minutes.

---

1. "I do not claim to be the author of this science of Osteopathy. No human hand framed its laws...." (A.T. Still, *Autobiography*, p. 302.)

The corrective principle in physiological biodynamics is more than mere exaggeration, direct action, opposing physiological action, et cetera. It is as Will Sutherland suggested when he was asked what to do with a convulsive case in a convulsive state: "Lock him up." Bring all the contributing factors present into the *Fulcrum*, from the ends of all the levers, into physiological biodynamic focus or balance. This is the point of physiological and pathophysiological efficiency. This is the point at which entropy can modify its dynamic.

More cases require the analysis and know-how of "lock him up" for effective treatment than the process of treatment to "free" the mechanism.

Lock them up: need to take disease/trauma pattern back to place of rest. (1984)

"Thank you for giving me the opportunity to watch you heal yourself." *A statement Dr. Becker would say to himself before treating a patient.*

"Normal" is a static term for values of health at a given moment. Man basically is evolving in anatomicophysiological functioning from his beginnings on Earth, through his birth and his walk about on Earth, to his final hours. His body is constantly modifying its structure-function towards improved survival and efficiency, even unto his last hours. The normal of yesterday is not the normal of today, nor will it be the normal of tomorrow. (1970)

Basic Energy versus Nervous Energy

A car can run without a battery provided you start it by pushing and get the generator to running, and drive fast enough to keep the generator going. But there is a danger you will burn out the generator.

Moral = You need a battery.

The conductor commands a sound image of the author's symphony to manifest itself. He expects the musicians in the orchestra to bring their living sound image from the manuscript of the author's symphony in response to the command. The Symphony of Life is reborn with onflowing LIFE.

Treat patient as a whole (Holy) person, regardless of what has been removed at previous surgeries.

The Whole Person. Everyone talks about it, but they don't do anything about it. Think BIG. (1974)

An observation: There is only one Authority within each of us, manifesting itself through our inherent mechanisms; and it is in all of us. (1980)

Tide = "Rocked by your inside cradle"

Healing can only take place in an atmosphere where there is no judgment.

I belong to that group of people who believe that "philosophy should be the precursor to action."

Running water finds its own way without strife.

✧ The unity of function includes power, matter, motion and time as a continuum. Function itself has a number of meanings from that of a normal or characteristic action of anything to a thing that depends on and varies with something else. We read in the word "function" more meanings than are given to us in a dictionary and rightly so. It is a word that has depth.

There is a similarity between the nature of the unity of function and the primary respiratory mechanism in that they cannot be accurately defined. As is true of the unity of function, the primary respiratory mechanism, too, is divided into component parts for descriptive purposes.

✧ Physician's role: He is a facilitator in a materialistic or mechanistic approach; he is a beholder watching It at work in a mystical or spiritual approach.

✧ "Life is a bunch of cells walking around with a common purpose."

✧ W.G. Sutherland: Natural forces are governing the mobility and motility of the craniosacral mechanism; that is the beauty of cranial treatment. (1981)

Tune to your Silent Partner, then to the Silent Partner of the patient, surrender and thereby become a participant in the process already going on.... The act of *surrendering* as a *participant* into the *unknown* does all the work. (1977)

The role of the physician is to serve man in whom health is made manifest. (2/10/1986)

The role of the physician is to serve man in whom Life is made manifest. (2/13/1986)

The role of the physician is to serve man in whom Life is present. (2/14 /1986)

The role of the physician is to serve man. (3/4/1986)

ONE-on-ONE relationship; not ONE-on-one (6/19/1978)
ONE-with-ONE relationship; not one-on-one (2/19/1981)

✧ The spiritual body is without problems. Tune into It, without concepts, as a beholder, watching It at work. Spirit does not correct the problem; spirit does not know the problem.

✧ You are getting back to Cause (W.G. Sutherland)
   Not a place, not a time, not a substance, not a mechanism, not a motion, not a concept. Be still.

✧ One-with-One, not one-on-one relationship

✧ The listening ear is the attitude in prayer and meditation—that we may hear, not that we be heard—only that we may receive impartations from within.

✧ God is individual selfhood.

✧ Goals are concepts:
- They are thoughts, plans, consideration.
- They are material.

Forget them, impersonalize them—God is not a concept.

✧ "Hear the Stillness" and Grace will flow.
Behold health delivering itself from within.
- Not the correction of overlying stress patterns.
- The Boss does not correct anything—It does not know error.

✧ The role of the physician is to "hear the stillness."

✧ To impersonalize your self leaves what? Stillness, Grace

To Know is to Be Still	Omniscience
To Be is to Be Still	Omnipresence
To Transmute is to Be Still	Omnipotence (1984)

I (CAUSE) am (effect)

I AM has ascendancy over the I, yet the I is a living part of the I AM. I AM is infinite; I is finite. I AM and I are inseparable (one) in their expression of life and living. I live for I AM. I AM expresses life through my living I. Therefore include I in all of my I AM meditation, mental activities, and manifesting action. In this LIGHT, there is no ego in I for I AM is my fulfillment. (1975)

19. GUIDING THOUGHTS

This is a selection of quotations and short articles that Dr. Becker
collected over the years. Items were chosen in order to help the reader
appreciate the influences on Dr. Becker's life and to see the origin of
some of his distinctive language. These items also reveal something of
Dr. Becker's nature and beliefs. References are given where they
existed or could be found.

OSTEOPATHY

Andrew Taylor Still

✧ Your osteopathic knowledge has surely taught you, that with an intimate acquaintance with the nerve and blood supply, you can arrive at a knowledge of the hidden cause of disease, and conduct your treatment to successful termination. This is not by your knowledge of chemistry, but by the absolute knowledge of what is in man. What is normal, and what abnormal, what is effect and how to find cause. (*Philosophy of Osteopathy*, p. 220)

✧ The most any Physician can do for a patient is to render operative the forces within the body itself.

✧ ...And after all our explorations, we have to decide that man is triune when complete. First the material body, second the spiritual being, third a being of mind which is far superior to all vital motions and material forms, whose duty is to wisely manage this great engine of life. (*Philosophy of Osteopathy*, p. 26)

✧ ...The student of any philosophy succeeds best by the more simple methods of reasoning. We reason for needed knowledge only, and should try and start out with as many known facts as possible.

✧ Principles to an Osteopath means a perfect plan and specification to build in form a house, an engine, a man, a world, or anything for an object or purpose. To comprehend this engine of life or man which is so constructed with all conveniences for which it was made, it is necessary to constantly keep the plan and specification before the mind, and in the mind, to such a degree that there is no lack of knowledge of the bearings and uses of all parts. (*Philosophy of Osteopathy*, p.19)

✧ Building and healthy renovation are united in a perpetual effort to construct and sustain purity. In these two are the facts and truth of life and health.

✧ The difficult part about osteopathy is acquiring the intimate knowledge and understanding of the structures and the fluid and forces that govern their action.

✧ We see in the fascia the framework of life, the dwelling place in which life sojourns. The fascia gives one of, if not the greatest problems to solve as to the part it takes in life and death.

✧ Let us not be governed today by what we did yesterday, nor tomorrow, but what we do today, and day by day we must show progress.

✧ Keeping in mind the osteopathic concept the human body does not function in separate units but only as a harmonious whole, and the fellow who masters it as such, will find that he is the specialist of all specialists and that is a life-time job of any man or woman.

✧ Nature never made a philosopher. She made man to learn and act. Man can make of himself a philosopher or a fool.

✧ Never surrender, but die in the last ditch. This is a war not for conquest, popularity, or power. It is an aggressive campaign for love, truth, and humanity.

✧ The science of Osteopathy is based on a system of reasoning that does not go beyond principles and truths that can be proven to exist in all of man's make-up—both physical and vital.

✧ Any variation from perfect health marks a degree of functional derangement in the physiological department of man.

✧ Any variation from health has a cause and the cause has a location. It is the business of the osteopath to locate and remove it (cause), doing away with the disease and getting health instead.

✧ The human body is a machine run by the unseen force called life, and that it may be run harmoniously it is necessary that there be liberty of blood, nerves, and arteries from the generating point to destination.

✧ Osteopathy to me has but one meaning, and that is that the plan and specification by which man is constructed and designed shows absolute perfection in all its parts and principles. When a competent anatomist (as the successful Osteopath must be), in treating the human body, follows this plan and specification, the result will be a restoration of physiological functioning from disease to health. ("Concerning Osteopathy," p. 36)

✧ An Osteopath is only a human engineer, who should understand all the laws governing his engine and thereby master disease. (*Autobiography*, p. 253)

Function is structure in action; structure is function after action.

                                       –Charles Bowles, D.O.

The basis of science is observation: by sight, by hearing, and by palpation.

      Sight can be shared,

      Hearing can be shared,

      Touch cannot be shared it is self taught.

                                       –Irvin Korr, Ph.D.

MEDICINE

THE ART OF THE practice of medicine is to be learned only by experience; 'tis not an inheritance; it cannot be revealed. Learn to see, learn to hear, learn to feel, learn to smell, and know that by practice alone can you become expert.

–Sir William Osler

What we call sense or wisdom is knowledge, ready for use, made effective, and bears the same relation to knowledge itself that bread does to wheat.

–Sir William Osler

Position follows motion as a shadow; motion is position on the run.
– Sir Charles Sherrington

You must always be students, learning and unlearning till your life's end, and if, gentlemen, you are not prepared to follow our profession in this spirit, I implore you to leave its ranks and betake yourself to some third-class trade.

–Joseph Lister

SCIENCE

THE MOST BEAUTIFUL THING we can experience is the mysterious. It is at the source of all true art and science.

–Albert Einstein

I have often had cause to feel that my hands are cleverer than my head. That is a crude way of characterizing the dialectics of experimentation. When it is going well, it is like a quiet conversation with Nature. One asks a question and gets an answer; then one asks the next question and gets the next answer. An experiment is a device to make Nature speak intelligibly. After that one has only to listen.

–George Ward

Engineering know-how is not a science—it's an art. Like any other art, it helps to have someone who already has mastered the art to show you how he does it, but that doesn't mean you then know how to do it. You still have to start from scratch and learn the art in your own personal style.

The great tragedy of Science—the slaying of a beautiful hypothesis by an ugly fact.

—Thomas Henry Huxley

As Buckminster Fuller describes it, "Synergy means behavior of whole systems unpredicted by the behavior of their parts taken separately." Although he calls it energetic geometry and experientially founded mathematics, some say this description could be applied to medicine.

There is a use of concepts which introduces a spurious multiplicity. For example the triad: structure-field-function ceases to burden the mind when seen as triple aspects of a single formative process.

—Lancelot Law Whyte
(*The Unitary Principle in Physics and Biology,* 1948)

It takes a lot of energy to make a transistor or vacuum tube work, but it takes only a minute amount of energy to direct that work.

A Knowing Universe Seeking to be Known

...If such questions arose in the days of absolute, classical science, how much more likely are they today when reality is no longer something separate from us to be contemplated externally, but an experience in which the observer is always necessarily involved. In physics of yore the experimenter could stand apart from the system under observation. Today every measurement disturbs the thing that is measured.... Perhaps what is needed is a kind of Bohrean complementarity of method, in which all of the methods that humanity has historically used to approach reality—scientific, philosophical, theological, aesthetic, even mystical—are used together in all of their vigor. Such a procedure would require minds willing to tolerate, or even enjoy, paradox, contradiction and antinomy, but such minds are already required by the Bohrean complementarity of contemporary physics. *Contraria sunt complementaria* was [Niels] Bohr's motto. He intended to tell us something about reality. (*Science News*, vol. 123)

NATURE

MIND CIRCUMSCRIBES ALL THINGS. In like manner it abolishes time and space. The influence of the senses have, in men, overpowered the thought to the degree that the walls of time and space have come to look solid, real, and insurmountable; and to speak with levity of these limits is, in the world, a sign of insanity. Yet time and space are but inverse measures of the power of mind. Man is capable of abolishing them both.

—Ralph Waldo Emerson

Beauty as we feel it is something indescribable: What it is or what it means can never be said.

—George Santayana

The Star Gazer

I go into space like a mountain does,
The rock of my roots gripping the ground,
The height of me there in the thin air.
My eyes are arrows going for stars.
I love the stars. I look long.
No matter how far the star from me
I can hold the star entirely
In my eye. It is in me.
Feeling the strength of the star there,

I ride the black vacuum between us,
And we can be one thing.
Thinking long on someone gone
Is not dissimilar. We move beyond
What we see from where we are.

—Anne Elizabeth Knowles

How Human Is Man

Life, as manifested through its instincts, demands a security guarantee from nature that is largely forthcoming. All the release mechanisms, the instinctive shorthand methods by which nature provides for organisms too simple to comprehend their environment, are based upon this guarantee.

The nineteenth century was amazed when it discovered these things, but wasps and migratory birds were not. They had an old contract, an old promise, never broken till man began to interfere with things, that nature, in degree, is steadfast and continuous. Her laws do not deviate, nor the seasons come and go too violently. There is change, but throughout the past life alters with the slow pace of geological epochs.... "Whatever interrupts the even flow and luxurious monotony of organic life," wrote Santayana, "is odious to the primeval animal."

– Loren Eiseley
(*The Firmament of Time*)

SPIRITUALITY

WHAT IS LIFE? WE think of life as a pulsation, a heart beat, a thing that is living when its heart is beating. The body manifests life; it is expressing life. But the expression of life, such as a lever working upon its fulcrum, is not the life which is expressed. It is the lever, but life and power are in the still fulcrum—not in that which moves—not in that which pulses. Our bodies do not live; they but express the life of our Source.

—Walter Russell

We are but the instruments or transparencies through which and as which the power can act, and act in proportion to our stillness and our quietness.

–Joel S. Goldsmith
(*The Mystical I*)

Understand–through the stillness,
Act–out of the stillness,
Conquer–in the stillness.

But how, then am I to love God? You must love Him as if He were a Non-God, a Non-Spirit, a Non-Person, a Non-Substance. Love Him simply as the One, the pure and absolute Unity in which there is no trace of Duality. And into this One, we must let ourselves fall continually from being into non-being. God helps us to do this.

Consciousness is not only a synonym for awareness, but much more: it is an established sense of awareness *without a process*.

–Joel S. Goldsmith
(*The Master Speaks*, p. 255)

The following quotations are likely from Joel S. Goldsmith.

✧ The truth is no individual has power, because "I" am all power, "I" am omnipotence. An individual has no power. You of yourself have no power. You can never direct power; you can never use power.

✧ When you know the secret of "I", you abide in stillness and let "I" do "its" work: not you–"I", that "I" that is in the midst of you.

✧ Once this truth has been unveiled for you, it will never be veiled again. You will never be able to go back to making concepts of God or looking for God to do something to the nothingness and nonpower of the world of effect. Always that smile will come to your lips, and the word "I" will come, and you will be at peace, you will be at rest. Then, in quietness and confidence, you can be a beholder of God in action. You do not impel It; you do not send It forth: in quietness and confidence, you become a beholder watching It at work.

GUIDANCE FOR LIVING

Ten New Positive Commandments

1. I shall cultivate an open mind. (A mind that comprehends)

2. I shall live above trifles. (The friction is in myself)

3. I shall put real content into my life each day. (We grow to look like the statues we carve)

4. I shall hold fast to my ideal. (The highest good of which I can conceive)

5. I shall keep busy at my highest natural level. (See, find, and release new power)

6. I shall cultivate the habit of reading with a purpose. (Growth)

7. I shall seek for, and find the power to overcome small grievances, self-praise, self-pity, small talk, and popular notions. (Overcome self-pity and the world is yours, with the fullness thereof)

8. I shall never lose faith in the person I might have been, nor confidence in my ability to become that person. (We are in a process of becoming what we will)

9. I shall seek beauty in life through an understanding and appreciation of the laws of the universe. (Feed my soul daily)

10. I shall cultivate simplicity and serve with humility. (Forget myself in the service of others)

...If you can trust yourself when all men doubt you,
    But make allowance for their doubting too:
...If you can dream—and not make dreams your master;
    If you can think—and not make thoughts your aim,
If you can meet with Triumph and Disaster
    And treat those two imposters just the same...

          —Excerpts from the poem "If" by Rudyard Kipling

Rules of Being Human

1. You will receive a body. You may like it or hate it, but it will be yours for the entire period this time around.

2. You will learn lessons. You are enrolled in a full-time informal school called life. Each day in this school you will have the opportunity to learn lessons. You may like the lessons or think them irrelevant and stupid.

3. There are no mistakes, only lessons. Growth is a process of trial and error experimentation. The "failed" experiments are as much a part of the process as the experiment that ultimately "works."

4. A lesson is repeated until it is learned. A lesson will be presented to you in various forms until you have learned it. When you have learned it, you can go on to the next lesson.

5. Learning lessons does not end. There is no part of life that does not contain its lessons. If you are alive, there are lessons to be learned.

6. "There" is no better than "here." When your "there" has become a "here," you will simply obtain another "there" that will, again, look better than "here."

7. Others are merely mirrors of you. You cannot love or hate something about another person unless it reflects to you something you love or hate about yourself.

8. What you make of your life is up to you. You have all the tools and resources you need. What you do with them is up to you. The choice is yours.

9. Your answers lie inside you. The answers to life's questions lie inside you. All you need to do is look, listen, and trust.

10. You will forget all this.

Skills for Living

What does it mean to be confused? People through time develop an environment that they feel comfortable in and learn to harmonize with. When for one reason or another, we "reach" into another environment which is founded on a different set of needs, we are no longer in harmony with our own world. That's not to say exposing ourselves to various environments will lead to disharmony in our lives. Only when we experience these other environments (worlds) and hold on to them, bringing those elements and principles into our established harmonious living space, do we disturb the harmony of both worlds. By being too personal in a foreign environment, we become confused because we no longer have a sense of WHO WE ARE. The harmony in exposing ourselves to different environments can exist if we participate as an impersonal observer and by not attaching ourselves to worlds we know very little about. When we attach ourselves to any form of security other then the acceptance of WHO WE ARE, it just becomes a matter of time before the human mind creates whatever illusion my be necessary to survive in an insecure world. Everything from a cell to a universe exists in harmony. By being in harmony with ourselves through "acceptance" and "objective observation" we can appreciate the beauty that exists in the world around us.

I believe that our own experience instructs us that the secret of Education lies in respecting the pupil. It is not for you to choose what he shall know, what he shall do. It is chosen and foreordained, and he only holds the key to his own secret. By your tampering and thwarting and too much governing, he may be hindered from his end and kept out of his own. Respect the child. Wait and see the new product of nature. Nature loves analogies, but not repetitions. Respect the child. Be not too much his parent. Trespass not on his solitude.

–Ralph Waldo Emerson

...So it is with conclusions [when writing]. There's a world of difference between merely stopping and really concluding. The writers who only know how to stop are the ones who produce 600 dull pages. They write away from the beginning, never quite knowing how to end it all. The writers who know how to conclude write toward the ending. When they get there, intuition says, "Stop." So they end.

—Rushworth M. Kidder

The true art of SILENCE at the right time is a wonderful thing to learn. Too many words upset the balance and more is lost than gained.

—Walter Russell

The Lost Art of Listening

Look into the average business school curriculum and you will generally find courses on effective communication; but rarely one on listening. Listening is not just a social grace, it is one of man's most critical living skills. It directly impacts on every aspect of life, from the workplace to the home. And yet, no one is ever taught how to listen.

Listening is the underdeveloped other half of talking. We've made the assumption that because most people hear reasonably well they are also listening. Hearing is a physical process; listening is mental and they're quite different.

The problem is that most of us have very well-developed skills at faking listening. We make eye contact, we nod at appropriate times, we agree with the talker, and we're *hearing* most of what he or she is saying, particularly the factual content. But facts alone rarely make up the complete message. The *idea* of what is being expressed, the underlying *theme* of the communication and its context are equally important and may even be more significant than the factual content. Analyzing these elements in a conversation takes real effort.

What can we do to become better listeners? First, resist the temptation to start preparing answers before the speaker finishes. This comes from the listener's assumption that he already knows what the speaker is saying "instead of looking for things that might be a bit different." Another technique is for the listener to clarify, as the conversation progresses, what has been heard. Though listeners are usually unaware of it, listening also involves seeing, paying attention to tone, posture, body posture language and other subtleties; good listening is actually hard work.

Patience and Courage

In spite of the stare of the wise and the world's derision,
dare travel the star-blazed road, dare follow the vision.

There is one form of hope which is never unwise and which certainly does not diminish with the increase of knowledge. In that form it changes its name and we call it patience.

—Bulwer-Lytton

There's no music in a "rest" but there's the making of music in it. And people are always missing that part of the life melody, always talking of perseverance and courage and fortitude; but in patience is the finest and worthiest part of fortitude, and the rarest, too.

—John Ruskin

Most men can be brave for ten minutes, an hour, two hours; but to be brave for five years at a stretch, when it is tiresome, when there is no apparent glory in it, takes some doing...

Courage is a myth. There is only faith and doubt. Nor have you cause to thank me. You owe me nothing. If what I do has merit, then mine is the debt to you.

BIBLIOGRAPHY

Books Cited

Becker, Rollin E. *Life in Motion: The Osteopathic Vision of Rollin E. Becker, D.O.* Edited by R.E. Brooks. Portland, Ore. Stillness Press, 1997. [2,4]

Bornemisza, Stephen. *The Unified System Concept of Nature.* 1955.

Carson, Rachel. *The Sea Around Us.* New York: Oxford University Press, 1951.

Davidson, Stephen M. *The Twig Unbent.* Phoenix: Practical Publications, 1989.

Eiseley, Loren. *The Firmament of Time.* London: V. Gollanez, 1960.

Goldsmith, Joel S. *The Master Speaks.* Secaucus, N.J. Citadel Press, 1963.

——. *The Mystical I.* New York: Harper & Row, 1971.

Krishnamurti, J. *Commentaries on Living,* 3rd series. 1960.

Magoun, Harold I., Sr., ed. *Osteopathy in the Cranial Field.* 1st ed. 1951. Reprint, Sutherland Cranial Teaching Foundation, 1997. [2]

——. *Osteopathy in the Cranial Field.* 3rd ed. 1966. Reprint, Sutherland Cranial Teaching Foundation and The Cranial Academy, 1993. [2,3]

Russell, Walter. *A New Concept of the Universe.* Revised ed. Swannanoa, Va. The University of Science and Philosophy, 1989.

Selye, Hans. *The Stress of Life.* Revised ed. New York: McGraw Hill, 1976.

Speransky, A.D. *A Basis for the Theory of Medicine.* Edited and translated by C.P. Dutt. New York: International Publishers, 1943.

Starcke, Walter. *The Gospel of Relativity.* New York: Harper & Row, 1973.

Still, Andrew T. *Autobiography of A.T. Still.* Revised ed. 1908. Reprint, Indianapolis: American Academy of Osteopathy, 1989. [1]

——. *Osteopathy: Research and Practice.* 1910. Reprint, Seattle: Eastland Press, 1992. [1]

——. *Philosophy of Osteopathy.* 1899. Reprint, Indianapolis: The American Academy of Osteopathy, 1986. [1]

——. *The Philosophy and Mechanical Principles of Osteopathy*. 1902. Reprint, Kirksville, Mo. Osteopathic Enterprises, 1986. [1]

Sutherland, William G. *The Cranial Bowl*. Reprint ed.1947. Reprint, The Cranial Academy, 1994. [3]

——. *Teachings in the Science of Osteopathy*. Edited by A.L. Wales. Fort Worth, Tex. Sutherland Cranial Teaching Foundation, 1990. [2]

Whyte, Lancelot L. *The Unitary Principle in Physics and Biology*. 1948.

Books available from:

1. The American Academy of Osteopathy, 3500 DePauw Blvd., Indianapolis, Indiana 46268. Phone: 317-879-1881.

2. The Sutherland Cranial Teaching Foundation, Inc., 4116 Hartwood Dr., Fort Worth, Texas 76109. Phone: 817-926-7705.

3. The Cranial Academy, 8606 Allisonville Rd., Indianapolis, Indiana 46250. Phone: 317-594-0411.

4. Stillness Press, LLC., PO Box 18054, Portland, Oregon 97214. Phone: 503-265-5002

ABOUT THE SUTHERLAND CRANIAL
TEACHING FOUNDATION, INC.

THE SUTHERLAND CRANIAL TEACHING FOUNDATION, Inc. is a not-for-profit organization established in 1953 by Dr. Sutherland and senior members of his teaching faculty. Dr. Sutherland conceived of the foundation as a way of providing a continuity for his teaching.

Dr. Sutherland was the first president of the foundation, and, since his death in 1954, there have been just four subsequent presidents, which has provided for a continuity in the organization's teaching program. The presidents who followed Dr. Sutherland were Howard Lippincott, D.O., Rollin E. Becker, D.O., John H. Harakal, D.O., F.A.A.O., and Michael P. Burruano, D.O., who has served as president since 1993.

The charter of the Sutherland Cranial Teaching Foundation calls for the organization to dedicate itself to educational activities. It specifically states its objective as using its resources to establish the principles of osteopathy in the cranial field as conceived and developed by William Garner Sutherland, to disseminate a general knowledge of these principles and the therapeutic indication for this approach to treatment, to encourage and assist physicians in osteopathy, and to stimulate continued study and greater proficiency on the part of those practicing osteopathy in the cranial field.

In its endeavor to carry out these objectives, the Sutherland Cranial Teaching Foundation supports research, produces publications, and offers both basic and continuing studies courses. As a not-for-profit educational foundation, it accepts charitable contributions to support its work of perpetuating and disseminating the teachings in the science of osteopathy as expanded by William Garner Sutherland, D.O. The current address of the Sutherland Cranial Teaching Foundation is 4116 Hartwood Dr., Fort Worth, Texas 76109.

er inspired her to pursue the study and practice
of osteopathy. She remained in contact with Dr. Becker during her
time in medical school, graduated in 1979, and in the next year took
her first formal course in osteopathy in the cranial field with the
Sutherland Cranial Teaching Foundation.

After completing a residency in physical medicine and rehabilita-
tion in 1982, she began her private practice in osteopathy the following year. She became a member of the board of trustees of the
Sutherland Cranial Teaching Foundation in 1988, and in that role has
continued to teach courses, develop teaching materials, and work on
publication projects.

Her initial editorial effort was to assist Dr. Anne Wales in the edit-
ing of *Teachings in the Science of Osteopathy* by William G. Sutherland,
D.O. She then edited *Life in Motion,* the first volume of the work of
Rollin E. Becker, D.O.

Dr. Brooks currently is in private practice in Portland, Oregon.

ORDERING INFORMATION

Order from:

BookMasters, Inc.
phone: 1-800-BOOKLOG (266-5564)
fax: 1-419-281-6883
e-mail: order@bookmaster.com
online: www.atlasbooks.com

For quantity purchases:

Stillness Press, LLC
PO Box 18054
Portland, Oregon 97218
phone/fax: 1-503-265-5002

Available in Europe from:

Osteopathic Supplies Limited
70, Belmont Road Hereford, HR2 7JW
England
phone: +44 (0)1432 263939
fax: +44 (0) 1432 344055
online: www.o-s-l.com